BEYOND

THE

CLITORIS

A Complete Pack of Womanhood

By

Mercedes Rowe Asamani

Published by **SHEREIGN CONCEPT**

Cover Design By Osupong Designs

Amazon E-Book Services & Editing by *The Sedi Group* (Wilson Ayinbangya Amooro) wilsonamooro@yahoo.com

Typesetting, Printing and Binding: Royal Media Investment Ltd.

For information or enquiries, please contact:

+233555386024

mercyasamani@yahoo.com

Blog: www.yaagh.com

ENDORSEMENTS

'I feel deeply honoured to have been called upon to endorse the Health   Aspects of Mercedes' book entitled, "BEYOND THE CLITORIS". That health must occupy centre-stage of women's daily lives cannot be over-emphasised. This book, with its well-researched contents, should motivate the reader to better explore their own bodies and I strongly recommend its use'

Dr. Kofi Adu- *qualified from the University of Ghana.*

Paediatrician, Founder/Director KAHL

UK

'*BEYOND THE CLITORIS*-offers a new vision to the struggling Young Ghanaian and/or African woman to know about her body, emotions, and societal norms as well as educate her to embrace her vulnerabilities and imperfections in order to become the Ideal Women Our Country needs!

I strongly recommend this book to be read by every girl or young lady (just like "courtesy for boys and girls"), as well as parents.

The Anatomy, Physiology and Pathophysiology aspects of womanhood which is often not taught unless one takes that course in a secondary or tertiary level is well explained in simple English for easy comprehension.'

Mercedes, You remind me of the Late Maya Angelou."

G. Amma Oduro Manu, *MSN, APRN, FNP-BC*

Board Certified Family Nurse

Practitioner at PrimaryOneHealth

Columbus, Ohio.

DEDICATION

This book is dedicated to a young girl who has been through the mill, known more pain than love, shown more love than given, searched tirelessly for love and inner peace. It is dedicated to a young but old soul who has been thrown at with lots of pain, disappointment, betrayal, and all that could get pillows soaked with streams of tears. It is dedicated to a young girl who gives all even when she has none, who looks past the hurdles to reach to her goals, who gets strengthened by hate from others and gets driven to succeed by opposition. I dedicate this book to myself especially when I am nearing my 23rd year on this earth- I dedicate it to me for never giving up and being optimistic of better things and days to come. I dedicate it to me for being there for myself even when no one was, for being my own father and mother and my own sibling. I dedicate this book to myself for rising above every hurdle. I am proud of who I am growing into. I am indeed my father's Son.

AKNOWLEDGEMENTS

I owe special thanks to the Almighty God who has kept me all these years and made this book possible. My sincere gratitude to several people who made it possible for me to complete this book in the face of several difficulties and other responsibilities especially to Abena Magis, Able Delalie, Anita Asante and Mrs. Grace Afia Larbi who made great contributions to this book- Thanks for supporting a fellow woman and ruling out the assertion that women are their own enemies. To Ama Duncan, thanks for every word of encouragement and to Mrs Rita Krampah, who was introduced to me by Ama Duncan, I'm grateful to you for your great counseling services.

To Lady Josephine Adwoa Fowaa who I affectionately call Nana Adwoa, I'm very grateful for every word of encouragement and financial support. I am grateful for your true kindness- you don't need to pretend to care because you truly care about me and support me and also not forgetting Mr. Emmanuel Effah who brought such blessings and great people into my life including Mr. Joe Anokye, the current Director General of the National Communications Authority, Nana Adwoa, Sister Nelly Debrah, Mame Yaa Akyaamah and other wonderful people. Mr. Effah, I am super grateful for everything- the fatherly care and financial support; May God really bless you. Mr. Anokye, words alone can never express my gratitude to you and the entire Mframak3se family.

Family is never always about those with whom you share the same blood- you have indeed shown me that some friends are more than family, to Anita Anyemi who's more than a sister to me, I say a very big thank you. To my awesome 2nd mother who is my aunt, Naachey Dode Akaabi, the Paramount Queen mother of the Awutu Traditional Area- Mum, may God bless you.

To Mr. Julian Mawusi Cobbinah, I'm grateful for everything- despite our differences, you have been a big advisory pillar and friend. You are one of the few who understand me so well. To my little mummy, Perpetual Lomokie Akwada, you have shown me the worth of true friendship- hate and rumours could never break us and I am very grateful. To Sika, Randa, Modesta, Ewurama, Mrs. Alomele, Nana Yaa, Rita Perbi, Rejoice Akrashie, Rhodalyn Eshun, Maame Saah, and all the ladies crew, I love and appreciate your support. To my pivot family: Richmond Asare Tinkaro, Harry Aboagye, George Sarpong, Mike Sarpong, Micheal Obiri Yeboah, Mandela Asafo-Adjei and the sweet girl, Ivy Vera Arhin- God bless you for everything. Aziz Lawal, Ferdinand Boakye, Ernest Ohene Kyei, Maame Awereba, Bridget Opoku who doubles as my roommate in school, Ewurama Dede, Angela, Penelope Tetteh, my Young African Women's Summit (YAWS) family and all others that time and space won't permit me to listen, I appreciate

And not forgetting haters, I'm grateful to you because you give me the urge reach higher and jump barriers. You inspire and motivate me to do better everyday. God bless you all.

TABLE OF CONTENTS

FOREWORD

BEYOND THE CLITORIS practically helps its reader to understand the intricacies of womanhood. The author uses her own experiences which are quite shocking at certain points, to illustrate her message.

It is a book for all: men and women, because indeed we all need to understand that there is much more to a woman than her Clitoris.

Ama Duncan

Founder of Corporate Training Solutions and The Fabulous Woman Network.

HOW THIS BOOK WAS WRITTEN AND WHY- by *Mercedes Rowe Asamani*

You might be wondering why this book was written and for what reason it was. The title might have already given you a gist of what the book entails except you are still wondering what a book with such a title will be about. I have always had the passion for womanhood and issues relating to womanhood ; gender equality issues, the societal perception of women, women and education, the influence of the society on womanhood, women and violence and every other issue relating to womanhood. I have for some time now been conducting courses on women related issues with some certificates in some courses. I have also studied a lot of materials online and learnt a lot from the experiences of others and this heightens my appetite for issues of womanhood daily.

Most men reduce women to just sex symbols; they only act with care and understanding in the bedroom to please themselves without considering what the woman might be going through, mentally. Beyond our clitoris , beyond our sexuality, lots of vital subjects shape and mould us to be the women that we are. Instead of being selfish and not asking questions, bear it in mind that our experiences, our biological make up, the environment and a whole lot process into the finished products we are. Most of you always say that the woman is complicated and difficult to please but I can tell you for a fact that the woman is the most understandable and simple. You just need to understand what womanhood simply is about and you are good to go. It's just like not knowing that most pregnant women nag; naturally you start complaining because you are oblivious to this fact. Have you ever asked yourself why your woman acts cold or gets angry easily or is materialistic or extravagant or doesn't love sex, is scared to show emotions, is prone to a particular disease and etc? Instead of running around complaining, sit her down and ask questions and I can tell you for a fact that when you are done listening to her, you will know the reason why she does certain things.

I, for instance, love spending money, a lot; I could spend a lot in a day and mostly not just on myself but friends as well, if I have much. Anyone from afar will never understand and probably call me a "show off" or insane especially when I even give my last money to someone while I starve but this is a habit I keep fighting myself over. I grew up in a rich home, daddy could afford giving me everything. When I was in boarding school, in the lower primary, daddy would buy me provisions and buy some for my friends who didn't have enough. He would visit me and give money to my friends and sometimes even pay for the excursion fees of some of my friends. Back in 2002, I received 100,000 Cedis or now 10 Ghana Cedis as weekly upkeep money, coupled with a lot of provisions; so I grew up spending a lot and giving out my last Cedi, even if it meant starvation. - Now things have changed and daddy is no more and I keep battling with myself to stop the habit of giving more than I have and spending more than I can afford, but someone somewhere won't seek the reason behind my actions but would rather jump straight into conclusion. Instead of judging people, ask questions.

I grew up living with one family friend or relative or another because daddy was always away doing business and mum was abroad. I grew up harboring a lot of pain and hurt in me because sometimes living with people deprives you from expressing your views freely. I spoke my all in school and came home with sealed lips and bottled up emotions. I couldn't share my pain with anyone, not even my first menstruation, because no one cared to listen and this experience has caused a lot of changes in my life. I went through series of sexual abuse but couldn't share because no one really had time for me. I'm still battling with my heart over a lot of issues and mostly keep my pain to myself and fight my fears alone because I feel no one cares to listen. I grew up hating sex because of the series of sexual abuse. My boyfriend jilted me because I told him I dislike sex. What if he had taken time off to ask why I thought and felt that way? He would have known my reasons and probably helped me but he thought I was selfish and just left. Instead of jumping into conclusion, just listen-it is not too difficult to listen. Most relationships, families, friendships and even marriages are tearing apart because we failed to listen. We can't be selfish in a world that involves others.

My personal experiences alone are long episodes enough to crave this love for issues surrounding womanhood. Experiences from my childhood till now are what give me the inspiration to write to empower other women. My experiences coupled with what I have learnt from authority or experts, traditions and culture, theories and literature and the experiences of others are the semen that formed this embryo. The journey of a woman through the opening of the vagina and down through the placenta and into the gloomy world where she mostly feels alone till her eternal rest never ceases since women are the breathe of humanity-without them but of course with the "complementation" of a man, the human race ceases. The eternal cyclical nature of womanhood is what brought this book to birth. The book touches on the totality of the woman from family, to health, to her society, to herself and also personal experiences of myself and ends with the contributions from other women on various issues relating to womanhood. It is a complete pack of what womanhood entails.

There is an Akan adage that says that, until the animals hunted by the hunter start writing their own history or stories, the hunter will always portray himself as the greatest and bravest. It is high time African women started defining womanhood by themselves-others have written our stories and portrayed us as the weak creatures because our long silence has given them the strength to define us. This book was written to define ourselves by ourselves because it is only she that wears her footwear that knows where it hurts most or knows where it nips and therefore it is only women that can tell well the feminine story. This book was written to touch on various issues surrounding womanhood. I always say that womanhood is a world on its own-; a world, few can travel through, survive and understand.

This book is in five parts The first part is titled, " THE OPENING OF THE VAGINA" with about five topics under discussion., The second is titled, "SOCIETAL CAVE" with about five topics under discussion as well, . The third part is titled, "THE WOMAN AND HER HEALTH" which discusses various health issues that affect the woman. The fourth part is titled, "YOU ARE ON YOUR OWN" which focuses on how the woman can develop herself with the last but not least part, titled, "CONTRIBUTIONS FROM OTHER WOMEN" Centered on various contributions from other African women just as the title suggests. Information in the book especially on the Part 3 which talks about Health have been well researched into from various online portals. I recommend this book for all men out there and not just women.

Let me be your tour guide as you take a revelatory walk on the path of womanhood.

SEVEN SUGGESTIONS ON HOW TO GET THE BEST OUT OF THE BOOK

1. If you want to make the best out of the book, you must be determined to work at bettering yourself. Until you yourself are ready to change certain things in your life to better yourself, no amount of words or long theories can change anything about you. If you aren't ready for that new and better you, opening up your skull to fix in motivational words and theories will never cause a change. Be the change you want to see. Be determined to work at bettering yourself in order to make the best or most out of it.

2. If you are really determined to make the best out of the book, please don't rush through the reading. Don't flip pages and skim like you do to any ordinary magazine. Instead, take your time and read thoroughly in order to digest everything well and take notice of every word. Missing a word might mean missing something very important that can contribute to you understanding the book well. Don't miss out on anything, read thoroughly.

3. To make the best out of the book, you must stop sparingly to think over what you have read, ask yourself some questions and relate whatever you have read to the realities of your life. Understand fully what you have read before you move on to the next step. You can't climb a staircase with a very heavy load at your back; you must wear off all misunderstandings, confusion and etc. by thinking thoroughly over what you have read to have full understanding of every text.

4. It will be very difficult to make the best out of issues if you don't see yourself in those issues. It's just like you listening to the story of a friend who probably may want you to sympathize with her. Until you see yourself in her shoes, you might never understand what she feels or what she is going through. If you really want to make the most out of the book, see yourself in the issues raised in the book and compare it to your personal experiences and that of others.

5. Your little cousin brought a mathematics assignment home and asked you to help her out., You had to lie to her that you were busy at that time and that you would help her later just so you could run to your shelf and search through it for your old and dirty mathematics text book. Were you not ashamed of yourself for lying to the little child? Were you not embarrassed for not being able to help at that very instant? You could have prevented this by taking your notes seriously and studying regularly to retain the knowledge. If you really want to make the best out

of the book, don't just dump the book after reading. Review each chapter bit by bit to remind yourself constantly of what you have read and like a mental sessions in the basic school class, you will finally be able to recite your times table off head.

6. You can read the book cover to cover, day by day and every time of your life but until you put life in the words of the book by applying what you have read, you will be doing a cos 90 work. A good warrior is never one who stays in the confines of his room to brag about his prowess by fighting with the air but a true warrior is one that gets on the battlefield and puts whatever he has practiced indoors to work by defeating his fears. Until you apply the theories of life by living it, you will be a walking dead.

7. We improve ourselves and learn more by sharing our experiences with others and teaching them what we know. In teaching and sharing experiences, we learn new things that will also add up to what we know to make us better. If you want to make the most out of the book, share with others what you have learnt coupled with your personal experiences. Be your own counselor and a counselor to others.

PART ONE

OPENING OF THE VAGINA.

Chapter One-

THE FIRST BLOOD.

1. She looked on with fear and squeezed her small body to the corner. She watched on as the door got slammed and the key turned. She knew what was going to happen next and her eyes shone in fury with her heart crying out in pain. Clothes kept flying about and she kept squeezing herself in the corner as if she wanted to vanish into the wall. For a minute, she wished she had some magical powers to vanish. She got awoken from her thoughts by a strong pull and there knelt the horrible creature who claims manhood. He tore her dress apart inspired by her tears and pleas and devoured her like a hungry lion. She lay on the blood-stained sheet and cursed her birth and her mum for marrying such a beast. He had forcibly stolen her virginity.

2. She looked on as he lowered her unto the bed. His eyes shone with love and her grips on him only showed that she was in a hurry to have him. She had long waited for the day when her sweetheart will eventually deflower her. She looked on with passion and kept wriggling her waist in the air to the tune of his thrusts.

3. Akosua came home in tears and run into her mother's arms. She kept sobbing even when her mother kept consoling her to stop. She finally was ready to let out the reason why she was in tears. "Mummy, my friends insulted and called me a fool because they claim I'm still a virgin at this age". Her mum hugged her tightly and told her, "My dear, everyone has their sole right to their sexuality. You choose when to have sex and whom to do that with. Virginity has no relationship with one's intelligence or capabilities." She hugged her mother and run off into her room happily.

WHAT DOES IT MEAN TO BE A VIRGIN?

Judging from the above three scenarios, we realize that Virginity is lost in different ways. Virginity is the state of never having had sexual intercourse therefore; a virgin is someone who hasn't had sex but "sex" is defined differently by different people. Most people think that losing one's virginity is to do with penis-in-vagina but that limits the definition. Per the definition of virginity, we realize that it is the state of never having had sexual intercourse and sexual intercourse entails a lot and not just penis-in-vagina intercourse. There are other forms of sex, thus oral sex and anal sex which fall under sexual intercourse and there are lesbians and gays who haven't indulged in penis-in-vagina intercourse but other forms of sex but think of themselves as virgins. Others also just stay in their room and masturbate with materials without necessarily having a penis-in-vagina intercourse but are not seen as virgins because all of such acts fall under sexual intercourse. Others also believe that consent defines virginity, thus if the intercourse is not consensual, it means one hasn't lost her virginity. So for example, being raped doesn't make one lose her virginity so these others will judge not the first scenario as a means of losing one's virginity. It makes defining virginity very complicated but as mentioned above, sexual intercourse is not limited to penis-in-vagina but other forms of sex as well. You figuring out if you count as a virgin or not are much less important than how you feel about you sexual experiences. Ask yourself if you are happy with the sexual experiences you have had or decided not to have? What can you do in the future to make sure your sexual decisions will make you happy and safe?

WHEN IS IT RIGHT TO START HAVING SEX?

First of all, we all are different people and we make our own choices; never worry too much about what the other people do. It is not advisable to submit to pressure to do something because the majority is doing it. Deciding to have sex for the first time is an important and personal decision. People think about a lot of things like religious, spiritual, cultural and moral beliefs; family and personal values; desire; friends' opinion as in the story in Scenario 3; love and/or relationships as in Scenario 2 and some sadly or unfortunately do not have the choice to decide on when and who to have sex for the first time with since they are raped like in Scenario 1. Whatever drives your decision to have sex; it's important to wait until you are very sure of your readiness to have sex.

The average age (according to several studies conducted) when people have sex for the first time is 17. About half of high school students have had penetrative sex. Our bodies mostly get developed around that stage and our sexual hormones increase so our urge for sex rises to its peak during this stage and it is therefore not surprising that most people have sex for the first time during senior high school level and also at the tertiary level. But one thing we must all know is to own our sexual right and not be pressured by anyone to have sex. Some people regret having sex after they break their virginity; meanwhile, to some, sex is overrated. If you started having sex and you want to stop, you definitely can. It is not compulsory to continue having sex always just because you started.

You are the only best person to determine when the right time to have sex is, judging from your beliefs, principles and etc but you surely must be ready by law and by mind. It is right that you engage in sex at an age where you can be able to handle any consequences that arise out of it.

WHAT'S A HYMEN?

The hymen is a thin fleshy tissue that stretches across part of the opening of the vagina. The hymen can be stretched open the first time a girl has vaginal sex which might cause some bleeding or pain. The hymen can never grow back once it has been stretched open no matter the vagina tightening pills or ointments one uses; once it's broken, it can never be repaired. Some cultures or people believe that a woman with a broken hymen is no longer a virgin but having a hymen is totally different from being a virgin. One's hymen can be broken through sporting activities, usage of tampon which is used during menstruation, riding a bicycle and other vigorous activities even without having vaginal sex. Some girls are even born with very little hymeneal tissue that it seems like it was never there.

DOES THE FIRST SEX HURT?

Some women have pain and bleeding during their first vaginal sex or fingers and objects inserted into their vagina. This is due to the tearing or stretching of the hymen. Some may feel more pain and bleed more than others since some naturally have more hymen than others. Some may have some few blood stains and others may bleed more. So, a woman's virginity cannot be determined by how much pain or blood there is because some naturally have very little hymen. If you constantly feel pains and bleed during every sexual intercourse, please talk to a doctor.

DOES THE PENIS ALWAYS FIT INTO THE VAGINA?

It is not always that the penis can fit into the vaginal during vaginal intercourse; very uncommon though. The vagina has elastic properties and stretches much longer and wider during sex and childbirth. The length of most vagina are between three and seven inches long. This usually depends on a woman's overall height and body size. Some women might have discomfort during vaginal sex if the penis goes very deep and touches her cervix or certain parts of her vagina and it is normal.

CAN ONE GET PREGNANT DURING THE FIRST TIME?

YES! Whenever semen or pre-cum gets on the vulva or in the vagina, one can get pregnant-whether it is the first time or the thousandth time. That's why it's advisable to use both birth control pills and condoms during sex, if one is not ready for pregnancy. The best contraception is abstinence. It is very advisable to abstain from sex until one is old enough to take up responsibilities.

VIRGINITY TEST.

A virginity test is the practice and process of determining whether a person, usually a woman is a virgin by testing for the presence of an intact hymen on the assumption that it can only be torn as a result of vaginal sex. Virginity test is widely considered as controversial, both because of its implications for the tested girls and because it is viewed as unethical. In cases of suspected rape or sexual abuse, a detailed examination of the hymen may be performed but the condition of the hymen alone is often inconclusive. Virginity is mostly tested by the insertion of a doctor's or an elderly woman's (mostly in some African culture) two fingers into the vagina to check the level of vaginal laxity. However, the usefulness of these criteria has been questioned by medical authorities and opponents of virginity testing because vaginal laxity and the absence of hymen can be caused by other factors.

Some cultures perform virginity tests to prove the Bride's virginity prior to her marriage and most doctors and opponents of vaginal testing see this as sexist and an abuse to women and denial of one's privacy. Most countries have banned this practice but the fact is that some cultures still encourage it despite the opposition.

I believe that everyone should have their own right over their sexuality without pressures from anyone including virginity testing.

RAPE

The term "rape" originates from the latin word, "rapere" which means to snatch, to grab, or to carry off. Rape is a type of sexual assault usually involving sexual intercourse or other forms of sexual penetration carried out against a person without that person's consent. The act may be carried out by physical force, coercion, abuse of authority or against a person who is incapable of giving valid consent; such as one who is unconscious, incapacitated, has an intellectual disability, or is below the legal age of consent. NO MEANS NO: respect the sexual preference of any woman, whoever she may be. This may sound controversial but it is equally rape to have forced sex with your wife. Everyone has their right to choose whom to have sex with and when to have sex so the sexual choices of others must be respected.

Report every rape case to the nearest police station without fears; report even if it is your father. If he look at you without pity to hurt you, you should never have pity for him when allowing him to face the law. Rape should not be settled at home with families taking money from culprits and letting it go. Please report all rape cases to the police stations for culprits to be arrested and charged to serve as a deterrent to other inhumane characters out there. Remember to report the victim to the nearest hospital for a medical check after a rape or defilement incident.

Anybody can be the culprit in a rape case so be careful who you trust. Even your own father can rape you but know that, no matter who the culprit is, it should not stop you from reporting him to the police. Culprits of rape are mostly unsuspecting- they are the people we mostly trust and we must report any sexual gestures from such people.

When we talk about rape or sexual abuse in general, the female gender mostly becomes our focus with less focus on the males. Meanwhile, these boys suffer silent sexual abuse. Some of them as early as age 8 get sexually abused by their step mothers, mothers' friends, cousins, sisters' friends and even peers etc. They keep it to themselves because same platform is not given when it comes to issues of sexual abuse. It's same with issues of domestic violence where attention is given to women victims than men, making it difficult for male victims to report. I have a couple of male friends who suffered sexual abuse at a tender age but couldn't ever speak about it. Let us give same platforms to our sons and brothers. Let us protect our boys too.

CHAPTER TWO-

THE FIRST CRY.

On that fateful night, the big balloon burst and instead of the usual chants of joy, it was a night of pain. After carrying it for nine good stress-filled months, her vagina was overstretched and she could no longer stand the pain so she gave out a loud cry that could be heard down the stairway and gave a deep sigh when she heard the tiny cry. The balloon had finally burst open and a pretty baby girl had come out. Tears of joy run down her mummy's eyes and she dozed off quietly with pursed lips as she heard cries from her new-born baby who was being whisked away by the midwives for bathing.

A baby is a blessing to a mother or the family and one must be delighted about her baby no matter the means by which she had her. Babies know no mistakes, troubles or shame and so pain must never be transferred from mothers to their children who never contributed to their fate. Not all children are born out of love but it is the responsibility of every mother to love their children no matter what. A friend of mine narrated to me her story about how she had her first and only son. She said,

"That late evening, I was returning from church when I realized that a particular guy has been following me from a particular junction after church. I started quickening my steps so that I can get off that lone path to a path where there were people around. I started running when I realized he had also increased his pace only to get stumbled over by a huge foot; I raised my head only to see another gentleman standing right before. I thought I had found my saviour and I sighed with relief only to hear another voice from behind asking him to carry me. I started screaming and crying as these guys carried me into a nearby uncompleted building. They covered my mouth with a rag and took turns in devouring me. While they took turns, they kept spewing insults at me that, "foolish girl, whenever you are passing by to church and we call you, you refuse to come. This is your punishment"

I then realized who they were; some two guys who always sat smoking on the football park close to the church. This incident changed my life; I was only 15 and a JHS3 student preparing for her Basic Education Certificate Examination (BECE) and here I was pregnant with no idea about who the father was. Attempts to arrest those guys proved futile because we never saw them again. I was lucky to have supportive parents who due to their religious stands rejected all suggestions of aborting the baby and so I sat for the BECE and passed successfully but I had to wait at home for a year to breastfeed my son before enrolling in the senior high.

19

It wasn't easy at all; the stigma from friends and even church members was frustrating. My parents had to relocate to save me the possibility of me being depressed or harboring suicidal thoughts. I even hated my son when he was born because I felt he put me through all this until I realized that my child had faulted not and it was my duty to love him unconditionally. I am now a successful accountant and I am proud of my son who has been my strength and we are the best of friends. I never regret having him as my son and I've grown past the horrible rape experience."

I shared this story so you will know that no matter the circumstances that led to you having your child, you should never hate the child because of those circumstances. This is a child who knows nothing about those experiences; instead of venting out your anger on him or her, please love them because it was out of your wombs they came. The placenta which held him to you is the bond that exists between you both and nothing should come in between you. You call that man who impregnated you silly because he shirked his responsibilities and so you hate his child, I mean the child you carried for nine months. And you have abandoned your child. Don't you think you are being double silly? We all make mistakes, get over it and love your child. Don't let him grow up into a bitter person because you will only be teaching him to do same to another's daughter if you raise him with hatred. Conditions shouldn't define your love for your child and that is why a mother's love is said to be unconditional. Some have grown into bitter, recalcitrant adults all because they were not given the needed love, care and attention. Don't raise a monster because hurt people, hurt people.

A friend shared his story of how his mother abandoned him after his birth all because she was angry about the fact that despite the many times she tried aborting her child, she never could. She was angry at herself and the stubborn foetus for refusing to be flushed out so she left him and went away after his birth. Now, this friend of mine has grown into a successful man and his mother is now pleading for forgiveness. He has shut his heart out and is not ready to forgive her but I only hope that he does that one day so he doesn't also end up raising his child in pain. Why should an irresponsible man, a failed contraception, an unplanned pregnancy, a failed abortion define your love for a baby you carried for nine months? Never let hatred consume you so much that it leads you to vent your anger and pain on innocent souls. It will only create a chain of pain and hatred and that can never bring peace in this world.

YOUR CHILD IS YOUR VERY OWN

"Move out of my husband's house if you can't comply with simple rules", these were words from a mother's mouth to her own daughter. Are you surprised? Her very own child!.

It gets surprising and saddening by the day but this is a canker destroying many mother-child relationships out there. There is a saying that if you love me, love my dog but it seems this saying is gradually dying off as most women are rather interested in getting rings on their fingers to be called wives and don't mind abandoning their children to run off with men or stay with them. While others deny to these men of ever having children, others are asked by these men to choose between being with them and their children and they gladly choose the men over their children; two selfish entities. If he truly loves you as he says he does, can he not accommodate your child- a fruit from your vagina, the very one he wants to enter? How can you abandon your child in the name of keeping a man?

I listened to a radio interview recently about a lady who was constantly raped by her step-father. Her mother whom she confided in asked her to keep it a secret so she doesn't ruin her marriage else she, the victimized lady will be thrown on the streets. This child has kept this a secret for fear of being thrown out and has had several abortions with her step-father and her mother being the one who even gives her the medication to flush the foetus out. I was caught in tears after hearing her story and I wondered if her mother was human or a beast. How can you sacrifice your daughter's life for marriage? Is she not the baby you carried in your womb for nine months? It is totally selfish for a mother to do this and has no justification for that. Don't tell me it's because the man takes care of you-so you no longer have the capability to work and in your quest to fill your belly and your sexual desire, you abandon your child?

Another woman also married for about five years without her husband ever knowing that she had a son. Her husband fortunately but unfortunately for her found out that she did have a son, five years into their marriage. Her biggest and only excuse was that, she thought the man would leave her if he had knowledge that she had a child so she gave her son to her accomplice, her mum, to be able to get married. The man after hearing this filed for a divorce and left the woman for good. How on earth can a mother abandon her child to be able to get the title, Mrs?

I remember vividly when my own mum told me that she doesn't want me close to her because I will destroy her marriage. She was happy abroad with husband and kids and saw me as a nuisance because I was from a different father. She could even tell me that she has other four kids and did not matter if I was not counted as her child. At that tender age, she could say all these hurtful things to me all because she was happy with another man and her justification was that I was stubborn. Ok, let's say I truly was stubborn; but did I ever deserve these words?

Mothers, future mothers, women, know that your child is your lifetime property. Your child is yours and you must love them unconditionally. A mother is never one who has given birth but a mother is one who can love unconditionally and protect a child. Some women have given birth but will never be called mothers, they will never be celebrated by their children, their children will never be proud of them because they have never been mothers but others will be called mothers because they understand motherhood. You loving unconditionally never means spoiling your child. If you love your child, you will correct them when they are wrong and never leave them astray but above all, you will love them no matter what and that is what makes a mother's love exceptional from all others. Guide your wards to make the right choices- Don't just be a bearer of a child, be a MOTHER.

DON'T LET OTHERS RUN YOUR MOTHER-CHILD RELATIONSHIP.

Show me a mother who has perfect children and I will show you a man who can see his back. There is no perfect relationship anywhere; even God has problems with man, always. Never be tempted to think that others have perfect children with perfect attitudes because they always tell you so to turn you against your children. Never compare your child to another; you can only be their guide and motivator to be the best children you want. Have you asked if the person turning you against your child has a perfect child? They may even be having children with the worst attitudes but might want to turn you against yours. Never allow people to run your family for you.

After my daddy died, my mother made me stay with a family friend and that was where my woes and troubles with my mum started. By then I was in the boarding house at a tender age due to the fact that my mother was abroad and my dad was a busy man. I was exposed to a lot and could do so many things on my own even at age 8. When daddy died, my mum took me away to live with a family friend who was a pastor and married with children. Life with them was at first very good, probably because I was new to them. At age 11, I was washing bails of clothes from the husband to the last child. My mother's friend, who was rather the man, kept complaining about how the woman mistreated me but she always threatened him with a divorce. I could wash bails of clothes even in the morning before leaving for school and get beaten with canes and belt hooks whenever I reported even a minute late to the house (I eventually stopped the boarding school).

I wasn't allowed to have friends and was beaten with a belt hook whenever a friend came to visit. My life was reduced to servitude at that tender age and I had no one to talk to. Whenever my mum called, I was made to stand right beside them to receive the call so that I could never complain to my mum; they rather kept spewing bad and untrue things about me to mum and as naive as my mother was, she believed them without ever listening to me. She would rather call and insult me after hearing their untrue stories about me and this kept messing up our mother-child relationship. If only my mum had taken time to listen to me, things would have been better; but I was never given the chance to explain myself. I was judged, always. During my long stay with this family, I was only judged and condemned and I was never happy. No one ever saw any good in me so I tried committing suicide about three times to end it all since no one really cared about me but somehow my desire to prove everyone wrong and succeed always gave me the strength to move on. Whenever my mother sent me stuffs ranging from clothes to food to toiletries and etc, I was never allowed to touch them. I could sleep on an empty stomach and sob in my pillow all night yet dress up beautifully on Sundays like a happy family and watch her smile beautifully at her husband's sermon. I sobbed within, the scars from the belt hook on my breasts, back and thighs were hidden under that beautiful church dress. Only God, that is if he ever existed then, could see my bleeding heart.

My mum never had the time to listen to me but rather allowed others run our relationship and that ruined our relationship. It is NOT ADVISABLE TO ALLOW OTHERS RUN YOUR MOTHER-CHILD RELATIONSHIP because no matter what or who your child is, she is still yours. Love her unconditionally.

HAVE CONTROL OVER YOUR WOMB.

You need not to hate an innocent child because you couldn't either abstain from sex or missed your period tracker. Please, have control over when and who to have your baby with so you don't ever regret having one. Unfortunately for those who may get pregnant from rape, they don't have control over when to have a baby, I believe everyone should have control. Some mothers grow up hating their children because they had them at a time when they were not ready; either financially unsound or with the wrong man or at the wrong time of their lives. Instead of cursing your children over your avoidable mistakes, please plan when and whom to have your children with. There are various forms of contraception methods out there you can use to have that control.

FAMILY PLANNING

It is the practice of controlling the number of children in a family and the interval of births, particularly by means of artificial contraception or voluntary sterilization. Family planning may involve consideration of the number of children a woman wishes to have, including the choice to have no children, as well as the age at which she wishes to have them. These matters are mostly influenced by external factors such as marital situation, career considerations, financial position,

23

and any disability that may affect one's ability to have children and raise them, health issues and many others.

If sexually active, family planning may involve the use of contraception and other techniques to control the timing of reproduction. Other techniques commonly used include sexuality education, prevention and management of sexually transmitted infections, pre-conception counseling and management and infertility management. Family planning is sometimes used as a synonym for access to and the use of contraception. However, it often involves methods and practices in addition to contraception. Additionally, there are many who might wish to use contraception but are not, necessarily, planning a family. E.g. Adolescents or adults. Family planning may encompass sterilization and abortion.

Therefore, family planning services are defined as "educational, comprehensive medical or social activities which enable individuals, including minors, to determine freely the number and spacing of their children and to select the means by which this may be achieved. Modern methods of family planning include birth control, assisted reproductive technology and family planning programs. The use of the modern methods of contraception is an important basis for improving the long-term health of adolescent girls. The United Nations Population Fund (UNFPA) says that, "contraceptives prevent unintended pregnancies, reduce the number of abortions and lower the incidence of death and disability related to complications of pregnancy and childbirth." They also state that, "if all women with an unmet need for contraceptives were able to use modern methods, an additional 24 million abortions (14 million of which would be unsafe), 6 million miscarriages, 70,000 maternal deaths and 500,000 infant deaths would be prevented".

There are a range of contraceptive methods, each with particular advantages and disadvantages. Behavioural methods to avoid pregnancy that involve vaginal intercourse include the withdrawal and calendar-based methods, which have little upfront cost and are readily available, but are much less effective in typical use than most other methods. Long-acting reversible contraceptive methods such as intrauterine device (IUD) and implant are highly effective and convenient, requiring little user action. When cost of failure is included, IUDs and vasectomy are much less costly than other methods. In addition to providing birth control, male and/or female condoms protect against Sexually Transmitted Infections. Surgical methods such as tubal ligation and vasectomy provide long term contraception for those who have completed their families.

SINGLE PARENTING.

A single parent is an uncoupled individual who shoulders most or all of the day to day responsibilities for raising a child or children. A mother is more often the primary caregiver in a single-parent family structure that has either arisen due to death of the partner, intentional artificial insemination, divorce, unplanned pregnancy or shirking of responsibilities by a partner, etc. while most single mothers arise out of these, some also choose to be single mothers. It has been statistically proven that the lack of social support for single mothers causes them to spiral into depression. Most single mothers go through financial hardships and receive low levels of social support and these sometimes in the long run affect the upbringing of their children. Most children due to the absence of love and security from the other partners thus their fathers end up having psycho-social issues. The mothers even sometimes suffer same fate. It is advisable that we appreciate and support single mothers to give the best of care to their children and as said earlier in the previous pages, we must be responsible for our choices in who we want to spend the rest of our lives with or have a child with to prevent more of such situations.

ABORTION.

Abortion is the deliberate termination of a human pregnancy or the removal of a foetus or embryo before it can survive outside the uterus, most often performed during the first 28 weeks of pregnancy. An abortion that occurs spontaneously is also known as miscarriage and one that is done purposely is called induced abortion. The word, abortion, is often used to mean only induced abortions. When allowed by law, abortion in the developed world is one of the safest procedures in medicine. Modern methods use medication or surgery for abortions. The drug, mifepristone in combination with misoprostol appears to be as safe and effective as surgery during the first and second trimester of pregnancy. Birth control, such as the pill or Intra-Uterine Devices (IUD) can be used immediately following abortion. When performed legally and safely, induced abortions do not increase the risk of long-term mental or physical problems.

In contrast, unsafe abortion kills millions of women daily. Unsafe abortion is defined by WHO as a procedure for terminating an unintended pregnancy carried out by persons lacking the necessary skills or in an environment that does not conform to minimum medical standards, or both. Approximately 21.2 million unsafe abortions occur each year in developing regions of the world and over 99% of all abortion-related deaths occur in developing countries. The World Health Organization (WHO) recommends safe and legal abortions to be available to all women. In some areas, abortion is legal only in specific cases such as rape, ectopic pregnancy, poverty, and risk to a woman's health or incest. There are debates in most places over the moral, ethical and legal issues of abortion.

The UN Millennium Development Goal (MDG) number 5 aims to reduce by three quarters the number of maternal deaths in the developing world. Without tackling the problems of unsafe abortion, MDG 5 will not be reached. In Ghana, abortion complications are a large contributor to maternal morbidity and mortality. According to the Ghana Medical Association, abortion is the leading cause of maternal mortality, accounting for 15-30% of maternal deaths. Further, for every woman who dies from an unsafe abortion, it is estimated that 15 suffer short and long-term morbidities. Currently in Ghana, abortion is a criminal offense regulated by Act 29, section 58 of the criminal code of 1960, amended by PNDC law 102 of 1985. However, section 2 of this law states abortion may be performed by a registered medical practitioner when;

The pregnancy is the result of rape or incest, to protect the mental or physical health of the mother, or when there is a malformation of the foetus. The government of Ghana has taken steps to mitigate the negative effects of unsafe abortion by developing a comprehensive reproductive health strategy that specifically addresses maternal morbidity and mortality associated with unsafe abortion. To ensure these providers have the skills necessary to perform the service, in 2009, Manual Vacuum Aspiration (MVA) was added to the national curriculum for midwifery education to train additional providers in this life-saving technique.

WHEN THE PARENT NEEDS PARENTING TOO.

I had no intention of adding this to this book until after speaking to my very good friend, Ferdi, as I call him. I was apparently speaking to him about certain issues I had with my mum and all of a sudden he asked, "Have you ever wondered that the parent also needs parenting too?" I kept quiet for a while and kept brooding over this statement of his. He used so many scenarios to explain to me why Parents need parenting too. Most at times, our mothers act in a certain manner towards us that we think they hate us and probably regret having us but have you ever tried to put your feet in their shoes?

Have you ever tried to weigh their experiences in the past and how that could be having an effect on their attitude today? Have you ever thought about the fact that your mother needs parenting too so she could act like a baby in the arms of her mother, shed tears, share her fears and be pampered out of the past haunting them? Instead of we seeing our mothers as super humans or gods, let us see them as humans like us who also have emotions, who sometimes need a shoulder to cry on, and above all the fact that they are also fallible.

Let us not be always hasty to judge but try to understand them sometimes just as we wish that they do same for us. Ferdi, to sum it all up said, "Life will be better, if the child acts like the child and the mother, a mother". That way, we can live a life without entangling emotions.

Mothers must also learn to treat their sons and daughters with equity; quit raising wicked and heartless men by scolding your son when he expresses emotions or shows too much love. Most of such boys are called, "kwadwo besia" all because he is emotional and shows love. Mothers, stop raising inhuman men! Purging of emotions is not just for a woman neither is love; stop defining a boy's wickedness as a good quality for becoming a hard and strong man-strength is never gained from hardheartedness. Let your sons love, cry, share their worries; give them listening ears like you will to your daughters. If you keep pushing them to store their pain and emotions since you think that is "hardness," you end up raising "animals". Treat both gender with equity. Give opportunities to both, let them share the household chores and climb high the academic and success ladder. Don't limit your daughter's success to marrying a rich man neither should you limit your son's success to making all the wealth and marrying a beautiful wife. Life goes beyond these. Guide them both with fairness and let them make the best out of life. Strength never comes from wickedness or hate but one's ability to love amidst all the pain.

CHAPTER THREE-

FROZEN EMOTIONS.

Life can never be a bed of roses; neither can its street be a carpet of gold. Just as we age from childhood into adulthood and then wither off in old age, so is the journey of life. At a point we crawl, we rise sometimes and we run too-all of these experiences are very necessary to give a better definition and appreciation of life. Chetan Bhagat once said,

"Disappointment will come when your effort does not give you the expected return-if things don't go as planned or if you face failure. Failure is extremely difficult to handle but those that do come out stronger. What did this failure teach me? is the question you will need to ask. You will feel miserable. You will want to quit, like I wanted to when nine publishers rejected my first book. Some kill themselves over low grades-how silly is that? But that is how much failure can hurt you. But it's life. If challenges could always be overcome, they would cease to be a challenge. And remember-if you are failing at something, that means you are at your limit or potential. And that's where you want to be. Disappointment's cousin is Frustration, the second storm. Have you ever been frustrated? It happens when things are stuck.

From traffic jams to getting that job you deserve, sometimes things take so long that you don't know if you chose the right goal.frustrations saps excitement and turns your initial energy into something negative, making you a bitter person. Remember, nothing is to be taken seriously. Frustration is a sign somewhere, you took it too seriously."

Chetan's words come to confirm the fact that life is never a bed of roses; neither is its street a carpet of gold. We fall to rise again knowing that a survivor and a conqueror is never one who runs from the battlefield but one who stays on to fight with the last drop of blood in her until she is declared the winner- now, that is the spirit of one who runs the race of life- no matter the storm she faces, she is never stopped by the storms of life. Instead of it stopping her, she runs in the direction of the storm like the maze runner till she completes the race and declared the winner. Let me share with you my story.

ICED UP.

I got to this chapter and got stuck for days. I left my laptop for days because reminiscing my past awoke a lot of emotions and tore open a lot of sores. It is never easy trusting the whole world with your private life and experiences known to you only but I'm writing this anyway because I want to motivate and help others out there who are going through similar experiences and feel all is lost. I write not to seek pity-hell no! Far from that. I am sharing with you the most delicate part of my life-I hope I can trust you with it and that you won't judge me or have a bad perception about me but will walk through my life with me hand in hand in understanding and love and you will get strengthened by this- I care less about what you think though, lol. I know after sharing this, it will awaken a lot of family issues and etc but I'm determined to face them all because when I said I was ready to help another victim out there, I meant it and I meant it in spite of the consequences. Most of what I will be writing is not known to anyone not even my mother who carried me for 9 good months but I share with you this day because I want to inspire you and urge you on. I will try as much as possible to make it chronological.

I was born out of a lovely relationship between my dad, Mr. Samuel Rowe Quaye Asamani, (may his soul rest in perfect peace). My dad was a successful businessman and a proud SantaClausian because he attended Adisadel College, lol. He was comfortable and his name was associated with kindness. I grew up with only blurry images of who my dad was because my grand-mother of blessed memory, Ama Serwaa, was the one who was taking care of me even after my mother travelled abroad at age 4.

I hadn't seen him but only had blurred pictures of him when I was very little but those around kept telling me evil stories about my father so that I wouldn't want to see him whenever I asked them about him. Although I was very little, I could tell they were lies. My sweet grand-mother died in 1999 and on the day she died, her ghost came to Kumasi to give me my favourite bread (the long white tea bread). Oh yes! You may not believe in ghosts but I saw one. That early morning, we were expecting her visit because she always came by during the weekend to give me my favourite bread and some foodstuff for the family. She finally arrived and she gave me my bread but unlike her, she asked that no one accompanied her to the lorry station. Few minutes after she left, we got a call from my aunt in my hometown, Agona-Asamang, in the Ashanti region, that my grand-mother had collapsed and died while sweeping. We were very surprised because she had just left our house. She couldn't have possibly completed the 3hour drive back to my hometown. Few months after my grand-mother's death, we went to church, as usual at the Kenyasi Presbyterian Church, and there and then, a new chapter of my life opened. Unknowing to my maternal uncle who I was staying with, my father's brother was also in that church. He saw me in church that day and called me and asked of my name (I didn't know who he was). He called my father to report to him that he had found me and that we lived very close (my grandma hid me from my dad because she didn't approve of their relationship as I as told and per law suits I saw).

Few weeks after, I was told that my father will be coming around and as usual they started telling me evil things about him that he's going to kill me if he sees me and so I shouldn't come out when he comes (this was in 2002). I was hidden in a big trunk-like suitcase called `potomanto' to prevent me from coming out, only for the families to surprisingly see me with their stunned eyes. (I had sneaked out of the trunk after I heard them constantly lying to my dad that I wasn't around). Blood is indeed thicker than water. I needed no one to tell me who my dad was, I run into his arms and we spoke at length. From that day, he kept visiting and showering me with love and for the first time, he organized a grand 8th birthday celebration for me. A month later, he came to inform my uncle that he wanted to take me to the boarding house and voila. I started schooling in Rev. John Teye Memorial Institute and left Kumasi to be with my dad in his house at Lartehbiokoshie, although I sometimes came to Kumasi for short holidays. I was my father's third daughter (he had no son) and he always called me his son- I remember when he bought me male panties (supporters) for school. While at my uncle's place, I was constantly sexually abused by my cousin at that tender age. My joy was short-lived when after a few days of illness, my dad died on January 10, 2003 (I hope I'm right with the date). After spending the best Christmas of my life with him and spending less than a year with him, death whisked him away.

I started facing life by myself after my father's death. I spent my last Christmas with him in his home in Denyame before his death though I was mostly with him in his home at Lartebiokoshie, situated around Radio Gold. After his death, his testament was read and a lot of controversies arose. I later left Rev. John Teye and was sent off to live with a family friend of my mum who was more of an uncle to me and a pastor in Adenta to continue schooling at Elim Cluster of Schools. At age 10 I was washing clothes of my uncle, his wife and their two kids. You can imagine the heap of clothes I was washing.

I was subjected to a lot of pain and mistreatment and was always blamed for everything even for having a car accident while on an errand for a neighbour. I was blamed for running errands for that neighbour even on the hospital bed, instead of asking how I was feeling. I grew up blaming myself for everything and thinking I wasn't good enough until I was able to finally part ways with my past. My `uncle' always had issues with his wife and she sometimes threatened to divorce him whenever he defended me on an issue that he finally eventually would give up on. He gave up on me. I was beaten mercilessly with a belt's hook at the slightest mistake. I could sometimes go to school with bruises all over my body. Remembering this stage of my life brings me a lot of pain and tears. I am even in tears now but I don't want to stop writing this. I want to write this to motivate you even if it will bring tears to my eyes. I even feared I had breast cancer because my `uncle' would use belt hook on my breasts. He was lashing just anywhere.

The atheists are free to doubt the existence of God but I believe that there is a supreme being out there who despite watched me go through all these gave me the strength to carry on. I tried committing suicide thrice while living with this family because it got to a time, I couldn't take it anymore. I had no one to talk to because I was not allowed to keep friends and I couldn't speak to my mum because whenever she called, I was made to stand right beside them to speak- my elder sister whom I thought would understand my pain watched on as they beat me. One fateful evening, after I had told my 'uncle' that I had seen my paternal uncle outside my school when I was accompanying my friend to trim her hair and that he had given me some money which I had already used up in school before coming back home for vacation. There was no way I could have told him earlier because throughout my two years in St. John's Grammar, I had just about five visits from them- I could sometimes beg friends' parents to sign for me during Parent Teacher Association (P.T.A) meetings to avoid being punished. He called my sister to come home and complained that I was at my bad acts again all because I had taken money from my paternal uncle (I know you are wondering what's actually wrong with taking money from your own uncle). He locked the door as usual and right in front of my sister and her fiance who is now her husband, I was asked to kneel and I was beaten mercilessly with a belt hook and cane at the same time all because my paternal uncle had given me money. My tears meant nothing to them not even my blood sister- I started hating her from that day but it is all in the past and we are cool.

That night, I took out a new shoe they had bought for me from the monthly allowances my mum used to send and took out that poisonous substance in it to drink and end it all. But my zeal to succeed someday and to shame the very people who treated me like I was less than human stopped me from doing this. I was beaten for every little mistake. My school closed at 3:30 and I was asked to get home by 4:00; if I got home even a minute after 4, I was beaten up. I couldn't attend extra classes and Saturday classes because of this even when I was in JHS 3. I was chosen to represent my school in a district spelling bee competition and these same people never allowed me to go. They never made me have friends and I never was allowed to engage in anything that will enhance my development because to them, I had a whole lot of chores at home to do. Amidst all these, I was the best female student in the BECE and the third best grade (you have no reason to fail. I would sometimes wash heaps of clothes in the morning before going to school which made me late most times. Whenever my mother sent me stuffs from abroad, I was never allowed to touch a thing. My uncle's wife will enjoy everything with her children and I had no reason to complain.

One time, some of my classmates followed me home because they said they didn't knew where I was living and for it had been long years of friendship so they wanted to. I kept trying to ask them not to follow me because I knew I would only be bringing trouble unto myself if they did. They never listened and did and after they left, I was left alone to dance to the music I had started playing. I was made to sleep on an empty stomach and beaten mercilessly-That day, I decided to kill myself with my pillow but the quest to succeed kept me alive. I went to school the next day with swollen eyelids, lips and marks all over my body and though I tried hiding it from my mates, they knew the reason. I grew up with a lot of pain in my heart-I had no one to share my situation with so I would just cry in my pillow and sleep praying that I would wake up in a different world but it never happened. I was pounding fufu one time and I mistakenly hit the pestle on my `uncle's' wife's hand and that day, to my surprise, she took the pestle, threw it at me and used it to hit my head and then she asked me to put my hand in the mortar so she hits me too and yes, she pounded my hands too. I was only 13, how strong and experienced was I in pounding fufu?

The maltreatment kept going on and on and I couldn't take it anymore so I started looking for my father's family since my mother never had the time to listen to me but judge me based on the nonsense they always told her about me. I called the home phone in my father's house in Denyame and I was told my step mother had moved out to a new house. Then I remembered that my paternal uncle had given me his number the day he passed by at my school. After calling him, he sent me my aunt who's the paramount queen mother in the Awutu Bereku Traditional Area's number and one hot afternoon after having saved enough for transportation, I run away from home (that was definitely not a home but a house) to my aunt's house at Kasoa-Bawjiase and she was so excited to see me. My paternal uncle all along in, my absence, had been overseeing the house my dad left for my sisters and I and had been taking rents from there so he was able topay my fees from that term and I went to school. My `uncle' never came to look for me after I ran away and no one cared until 7 months after on 15th July when my `uncle' came to visit me in my school, St. John's Grammar School , to my surprise it was because my mum had sent him there to speak to me since it was my birthday. I won't even be surprised if my mum never knew I had run away from home because she didn't ask about that. Neither my mum nor anyone had been told that I even had a car accident when I was 10 and I was operated on until I told her recently.

I was very happy at my aunt's place and my step mother who was the then District Director of Education at Jachie and my step sister who was and is still a housemistress at St. Louis suggested that I transfer to St. Louis senior high since I had a good grade and they wanted me close as directed by my paternal uncle. I was reluctant to because I had gotten used to my school. During one vacation, I was asked by my mum to go to my paternal uncle in Kumasi for something she had sent. Unknowing to me, my `uncle' had fed her with untrue things about me and he had connived with her to send me to my paternal uncle in Kumasi to school there. She gave my paternal uncle strict instructions that he shouldn't take me to St. Louis or any Grade A school but rather to a school in a remote area so that I learn my lessons (I never knew what I had done to be learning lessons because despite the pain they put me through. I was still a very good girl but my `uncle' fed her bad news about me that I was a very bad girl and that he couldn't handle me anymore. Meanwhile, as young as I was in school as at 15, I had formed a youth advocacy group with my friends called "Voices of the Youth" and were all over the place seeking funds-the idea got stolen finally by some investment company who decided to help us and since we had no voice then, we let go but here I was, painted black to my mum and she saw no good in me and she never took time to speak to me either. My `uncle' had used me to cover up all the bad things he put me through).

I finally got to Kumasi only to be told that I'm no more going back to school in Accra and my mother had asked them to take me to Antoa senior high school as a day-student. I was so shattered that I decided to stop schooling but I remembered that I had come a long way to quit. I went to a school I never dreamt of attending and started totally new electives in from three. While I read literature, music, government and Christian Religious Studies (CRS) in St. John's Grammar for a year, I started reading economics, geography, elective mathematics and government in Antoa in form three. I registered for Nov/Dec in form 3 with the courses I read for a year in St. John's grammar thus CRS, government, literature and economics (I didn't register music because we hadn't gotten anywhere. I registered economics though I didn't read economics- I loved economics so while in St. Johns. I used to take my friends `notes and read on my own). I sat for papers I had read for just a year and one which I was never taught-it was definitely not easy but I wanted a way out of Antoa and so wanted to pass and quit. I had aggregate 15 and that definitely wasn't what I was looking for because I wanted to read law. I had no other choice than to accept my fate and stay there; most of my teachers were very supportive and my headmaster then. Mr. Frederick Addae, brought out the best in me. I started engaging in school activities. I was made the SRC secretary and I reformed the Writers' and Debaters' club of which I became the president. I took the school to district debate competitions and for the first time, they placed 2nd with a slight difference between Adventist girls' SHS and us. That day began my new joyful chapter- after the debate I still feel cheated, the chairman called me and congratulated me that I did so well and that we actually won and were supposed to represent the district but since we didn't have a strong debate club and other factors which they consider, they had to pass the win to the other school. He urged me never to give up and his words gingered me to move on up. I kept leading the debate team and the writing team too. I became the heroine of the school. In 2012, the Ashanti Regional SRC organized a regional essay competition and together with two other students, I represented Antoa. Amidst all the other so called `Grade A' schools, I came 2nd to an Asanteman High School student (nothing must stop you in your tracks not even your geographical location).

I remember vividly the day we were supposed to write the quiz at Kumasi Anglican SHS-the moment I entered in my Antoa senior high uniform, the first comment I heard was, "what is Antoa too doing here?" I felt sad within but that pain gingered me on to excel to prove everyone wrong and here I was receiving all the attributes from the then Regional Director of Education who was awed about the fact that, a student from Antoa senior high could actually come 2nd. He dashed me some money that day and one of the members of the Association of Past Executive Committee, Austin, asked that I join APEC after I'm done with school. I had earlier picked a form to contest the regional SRC secretary position which I knew I could have won but when it got to the day of congress, my uncle refused to allow me go with the excuse that my mum said he shouldn't. My mum and sister killed yet another dream of mine to be the Ashanti Regional SRC secretary. I cried my head out that day that I had once again been denied my dream.

Few months after staying with my uncle, things started getting tough there too. I was never allowed to speak to anyone and every boy I was seen talking was said to be my boyfriend and was beaten up with no explanation. My uncle told me his wife was complaining about the amount of money he was giving me, his wife also showed him a gift I had bought for a friend and so from there, he reduced the amount of money he was giving me for school. I could sometimes walk from Kenyasi to Antoa and that is about 5 km, and back, just to save some money for food. I mostly depended on my economics teacher, Mr. Frank Assuah, for money. When I got home late too from walking those dusty kilometres, I was insulted for being lazy and intentionally coming late. Life there was rough and smooth-it sometimes got better and sometimes very worse till I finally completed school. I asked for permission from my mother to be able to work to earn something for myself-growing up, I had always done things for myself. I worked for about two months and my uncle reported me to my mum that I had grown pompous since I started work and wasn't coming home early and not eating from home. My mum without listening to me asked me to stop working and I tried explaining to her that I just can't quit until I tell my manageress and wait for month ending but my mum sent my uncle to the office and spoke to my boss in a very bad manner. She had no reason than to let me go in pain. I angrily left my paternal uncle's house and went to my maternal uncle's house (the one with whom I was with during childhood).

I bought awaiting forms and had admission to KNUST to read Political Studies and told my paternal uncle since he was in charge of my father's house but he refused to pay my fees. My mum refused to pay too because she was angry about the fact that I had left my uncle's house. I went back to my aunt in Kasoa-Bawjiase to complain to her about my uncle's attitude. I spoke to one lawyer Osborn who was an APEC member and decided to help me for free to regain my father's house and get my mother to perform her responsibilities. The lawyer called my paternal uncle to schedule a meeting with him at his chambers in Adum. My uncle reported me to my mum and sent her the lawyer's number only for my mum to call and insult the lawyer. The lawyer called later expressing his disappointment and asked me if I still wanted to continue with the case and I said No and thanked him. Fast-forward, my late father's friend, called to speak to me and asked me to return to Kumasi. I did and went back to my uncle's house. A year later, I gained admission into the university of Cape Coast and my uncle delayed in paying my fees (because he was still angry that I had involved a lawyer) under the excuse the monies he had been collecting all along for years was used for maintenance and that he had no money for me (surprising right?). I kept my cool-my mum couldn't have done much to help because she had been down with stroke in the UK and was now recovering (she hadn't being helping exceptionally anyway because she knew my uncle was in charge of my father's house). I ran to my daddy's friend for help- already, he started making sexual advances at me after he convinced me to come to Kumasi and so I stopped my regular visits to his place-I needed his help now and had no other choice than to go to him. He ended up forcibly sleeping with me, my second abuse; and tried to do it again but never succeeded whenever I decided to run to him for help until I cut ties with him totally.

I finally got into school and I still am in school. My uncle keeps repeating the same line, "I used the money for maintenance" whenever I ask him for my fees he actually writes down every cedi he gives me and takes it from the rent whenever he goes for it. I've managed to pay my school fees and hostel fees myself and once a while I get refunded when he decides to finally give me a part of what he doesn't know I've paid. My mum sends me some money occasionally. I have come this far on my own; I am a fighter and I strive to earn whatever I want. One principle I have learnt to live by is never to remove my pants for a favour, never! I love to give no matter how little I have; I have actually paid a friend's fees for her before when I hadn't paid mine and this attitude of mine has never made me lack-I equally get people helping me without condition. There is power in giving and I will urge you to give wholeheartedly no matter how little you have. I have had to pay my fees by myself but my aunt, Naachey Dode Akaabi has been very supportive together with other friends and family. I doubt my mum knows even the level or the course I'm reading in school. I doubt she and my uncle know that I already have a book to my credit, that I have a foundation, that I write or blog. I doubt they know anything about me and I pray they don't even miss my graduation day. I am my own mother, father and sibling. I wake up each day thinking of my next meal, my fees, my books, working hard to earn something for myself and striving to develop myself meanwhile, there's a mother out there who feels she has 5 kids and so losing me won't mean anything, there's an uncle out there who has taken over and using what is duly mine and there are wicked family members of my dad out there who are busily fighting to take over what is mine and care less how I survive but hey, life is individualistic-we fight our own battles and win or lose them so I am fighting mine with or without them.

I have always been on my own, taken my own decisions, spoken to myself, committed mistakes and learnt from them myself. It has always being me, alone. While people had family visiting them in SHS, I was left to myself-I had to beg friends' parents to sign for me during PTA meetings. While others went to the university on the first day with their family, I came alone, when I fall ill; I lie on my hospital bed alone with no one to ever call to even find out if I am fine. I was robbed, I called home and I was blamed and insulted. It has always been me and me alone. While people receive awards and launch their books with their families present, I did these alone but I am not perturbed because I have to come to accept that we are fighting individual battles in life and that life is about ME, MYSELF and I, YOU, YOURSELF and YOU. When you learn to accept that, you won't expect too much from people and you will never be surprised about anything. Fight on till you reach the ultimate. Never say never!

Today, my mum and I are ok and she is trying her possible best to stay close all because she sees the strong and focused me who never gave up and she is proud of who I've grown up to become and I love her so much despite everything. I believe everything happens for a reason and I have been through all these because the experiences have made me stronger, more focused, and confident and determined to succeed. I have learnt to work and earn money on my own by making use of my God-given talents and hard work coupled with a good attitude. God has also been super good to me to draw into my life great people to guide and help me and I am currently doing a lot for myself and others. Don't think that I have arrived because I haven't- though I am not where I want to be, I take encouragement and delight in the fact that I am not where I used to be.

In all of these too, I have become a very hardworking young woman- doing home chores, vigorous work do not give me headaches because I grew up doing them. It has made me a good home manager amongst others and that's why I would always say that everything happens for a reason and it is up to us to turn stones into gold.

This is to tell you that, experiences are a two-way street and you either choose to be a slave to them or rise above them to rule and I have chosen the glorious path and that is to rise above them and have control of my present if I want to attain my desirable future. Take a cue from this and know that, we can achieve anything in life if we set our minds to it. All in all, I'm grateful to everyone because they unearthed the strong woman in me and made me who I am today. I want to be an inspiration one day- I want to hear people say someday that "if she could make it, I can".

CHAPTER FOUR-

WHEN THE ICE MELTS

Our experiences mostly shape and mould us-we are mostly what we have been through. Most people act the way they do because of their experiences. Our past experiences shape our behaviour and personality. I will start this chapter by sharing Hanan Parvez's piece on experiences and how they shape us. Hanan Parvez says that our beliefs and needs are the strongest factors that govern our behaviour. It ultimately comes down to beliefs because a need is also a belief- a belief that we lack something. When we were born, we were almost a clean slate-ready to collect information from our environment and form beliefs based on that information. He says that if you have carefully observed a child grow then you know what he's talking about. A child absorbs information from its environment so fast and at such a high rate by age 6, thousands of beliefs are already formed in its mind-beliefs that will help the kid interact with the world.

The belief we form in our childhood and early teens form our core beliefs. They are the strongest factors that influence our personality but that doesn't mean we are stuck with them. They are hard to change but not impossible. The beliefs that we form later on in life are comparatively less rigid and can be changed without much effort. Your inner child is still affecting your behaviour much more powerfully than you think! I personally don't drink alcohol because growing up, I was made to believe that it was harmful and so I am still stuck by that. I was prepared to keep my virginity till I got married to whomever because I grew up in the belief that, that was ideal but I had no power over that especially when I was sexually abused even before I could decide when to have sex. This inner child kept haunting me because it made me hate sex and men even after I willingly had sex with my first boyfriend in my adulthood, I started drifting away from him because I began hating him after the sex-yes, my past experiences were gradually shaping me and I had no power over it but hey, though hard, it is never impossible.

CHANGING THE BELIEFS

Hanan goes on to say that, the first step to change our beliefs is to become conscious of the beliefs that are shaping our personality. Once we have identified them, we need to dig into our past and understand why we formed these beliefs and now, this is the hard part. The process of formation of belief happens unconsciously and that's why we feel powerless before them but once we make the unconscious conscious, we start gaining real power.

Identifying the beliefs that we want to change and understanding how we formed them is enough for us to break free from their clutch and not let them control our behaviour. Awareness is like a fire which melts away everything. Try understanding it this way; suppose your job performance was very bad this month and your boss is disappointed in you. He wants you to make amends in the coming month but he doesn't give you any performance report and doesn't point out in any way what needs to be fixed. Will you be able to fix anything if you don't know what went wrong? Absolutely not! You need to know what went wrong in order to fix it. In addition to that, you need to know how and why it went wrong. It is same in the case with human behaviour- until you understand the underlying mechanism of your behaviour, you won't be able change it. I have already given you some personal examples but these are some examples cited by Hanan;

1. A child who was abused forms a belief that he is less worthy than others because of the way he was treated. So he is very likely to have a low self-esteem and live with shame for the rest of his life. He may therefore become a shy person.

2. The youngest child in a family receives a lot of attention from everyone around him and so he develops a need to always be in the centre of attention. As an adult, he may become a very showy, successful or a famous person just to remain in the centre of attention.

3. A girl whose father abandoned her and her mother may form a belief that men cannot be trusted. So, as an adult, she might find it very hard to trust any man and may have problems forming an intimate relationship with a guy. She might end up sabotaging every relationship she gets into without knowing why.

4. A boy who always felt financially insecure as a child because his parents always worried about money may develop a strong need to become rich. He may become very ambitious and competitive. If he fails to meet his financial goals, he may become severely depressed.

5. A kid who was bullied in school may develop a need to become strong and therefore he might become very interested in body building. If you interviewed gym addicts, you will find that most of them were either bullied as kids or were involved in a physical fight before. Very few do it just to improve their body-image.

Because of the experiences that people go through in life, they develop certain deep-seated beliefs, needs and ways of thinking. In order to fulfil their needs, they develop certain personality traits. They might not be aware why they have certain personality traits but their minds are working continuously in the background continually seeking ways to satisfy its needs. Contrary to popular belief, we can train ourselves to develop any kind of personality that we want. You might like some of the personality traits that your past has bestowed upon you but you can always change the ones you don't like by changing the beliefs that are associated with those traits.

Due to the fact that I lacked love, care and attention while growing up, I fell for every signal of these from the opposite sex and thought they loved me-I grew up trusting and befriending male friends rather than female because of the bad experiences I had with women. I entered some relationships to quit later after realizing those guys had just hit on my weakness thus my quest for love, care and attention-that's how bad our past experiences can shape us but through it all, I have recovered and I am gradually coming out as a stronger person.

CHAPTER FIVE-

MATTERS OF THE HEART.

Our heart runs our life and we cannot discuss issues relating to us without talking about our matters of the heart. The heart sometimes brings us pain and also joy-I choose to call it a double edged sword. Be very careful about how you treat matters of the heart because as Dianna Hardy once said, "everything that matters hurt until it doesn't matter anymore. Issues of love, sex, family, friendship, relationship and marriage are all matters of the heart and one must not be in it to fool the other because matters of the heart are never Child's play. Don't be the reason why someone's life ends, or gets shattered or gets destroyed. I pray you take a cue from the words of JoyBell C. She said,

"The only prescription for morality is this: Remember that every woman could have been your mother, every girl could have been your daughter. Remember that every man could have been your father; every boy could be your son. When it comes to matters of the heart, that's all that needs to be kept in mind, always, at all times. Whatever form of hurt you cause will echo in your children one day. Whatever form of judgement you make, must be held up against the condition of your father or your mother. When this is done-one sees that there is no room to judge and that there is no room to hurt another".

Not all of us will be lucky to find love-while we may love others who love us not; others may be so much in love with us but never thought off. While we may be scared to open up our heart to others, others equally are and it gets sadder and more confusing when we only end up falling for those who have already been taken. Whatever situation we find ourselves, know that love just like life and any other thing has a life span and we must get the best out of it while it lasts even if it means loving just ourselves. Overlook the boundaries, just imagine a world just for you or the two of you-whether taken or not, enjoy love till it catches expiry. A heart without love is a hurting and weary one- a heart with love equally hurts, so either choose bitter-bitter or bitter-sweet. But whatever the case, Love yourself.

LOVE

A portion of Tracy Chapman's song, "Matters of the heart" says,

`I can't believe it's so hard to find someone to give affection to and from whom you can receive. I guess it's just the draw of the cards in matters of the heart". If it is indeed the draw of cards then one definitely knows not what card the other is holding or what they are going to draw or even who will win at the end. In the game of cards, until all cards are drawn, you never know the cards each person had so it is in love- until all intentions are known, you never know the true feeling of the other. Actions speak louder in matters of the heart. Instead of re-echoing your love for others and trying so hard to convince them with words, show it. Love is shown not said. What then is love? I sometimes see love as getting something we never had from another and in this case; our experiences are likely to shape this. I have heard some women fall in love with guys or conclude that some guys love them because those guys were showering them with gifts and money when they had none. Most at times, we judge such women as being materialistic and not truly loving but I can tell you for a fact that, that is indeed love. At that point of their lives, probably what they needed most was someone to take care of their needs and so when they find that, they see that as love and love back.

Others also fall in love with guys because as at that point in their lives, they needed someone to give them attention, care and love and if they are able to get these, they end up believing those guys love them and they love them back. Others may also be looking for someone who will give them listening ears and comfort them and they also end up in that same cycle of love. Others may probably be bored and need someone to hang out with or someone who shares common interests with them-when they find these in others, they see that as love and end up falling in love and etc. This is to say that we should never judge the reasons some give for falling in love with others because everyone has a genuine reason why they do. I still stand by my words that I sometimes see love as receiving something we have always yearned for from another and we getting emotionally attached to them because of that.

Some also are of the view that love is a decision to be with someone. Wikipedia defines love as an emotion of a strong attraction and personal attachment. It can also be a virtue representing human kindness, compassion and affection-"the unselfish loyal and benevolent concern for the good of another. Ancient Greeks identified four forms of love: kinship or familiarity (storge), friendship (philia), sexual and/or romantic desire (eros) and self-emptying or divine love (agape). I will focus more on eros or romantic relationships since most see them as the most meaningful element in our lives, providing a source of deep fulfillment.

ROMANTIC RELATIONSHIP.

An intimate relationship is one in which you can truly be yourself with someone who you respect and are respected in return. It is an emotional connection that can also be physical. It is not always sexual- sex is a bonus in an intimate relationship. It should never be the basis for the start of a relationship. You can love someone intimately without necessarily having sex. Sex is an individualistic decision that must be ventured into only when one is ready and willing. Many people think that intimate means being physically intimate such as being in a sexual relationship. However, an intimate relationship can be with anyone who you are really close to and with whom you can completely open up to and be honest with. Intimate relationships afford you the opportunity to grow as an individual.

Now let's talk about romantic relationships, which unfortunately are not always intimate relationships. In a healthy romantic relationship, both partners respect each other and have their own identity. Each partner is an entire individual, not simply part of a couple. Just as peer pressure can negatively impact a friendship, partners can overpower each other and create instability in a romantic relationship. Romantic love mostly exists between couples and is distinct from intimate relationships. It is mostly sexual and a strong bond between couples but as said earlier, it is unfortunate that most romantic relationships are not even intimate. For some, it is all about flaunting someone as your girlfriend or boyfriend or having sex with someone with no intimacy. Most romantic relationships break up daily and encounter problems due to lack of intimacy. Most partners even end up cheating with the next person who provides them with that intimacy they lack and seek.

How can you claim to be in a relationship with someone when there is no effective communication between you two, ; when the other person knows you not, your fears, your joy and your pain, when you are faking a lifestyle to please the other, when you can't share your problems with your partner? In fact, the only thing that binds you two is sex and money and gifts- intimacy is definitely lost in such a relationship and the moment you run out of money to buy those gifts or go bad at your sex games, everything comes crushing. Most people have decided to stay out of romantic relationships and rather opt for an intimate relationship with that one person who hears them out and provide them with all the intimacy and will rather have sex with such people with whom they have this connection without necessarily having a romantic relationship with them. It is called, "Friends with benefit". I personally don't think it's healthy because emotions sometimes set in and friendships get destroyed. One must rather have a romantic relationship with someone they share intimacy with- date your best friend.

KEY PRINCIPLES TO A SUCCESSFUL RELATIONSHIP.

When intimacy vanishes from a relationship, the soul of the relationship dies- intimacy is the breath of every relationship. Don't just occupy space or flaunt the title of being her man or his woman; act it. It takes a lot to come by someone who can love and accept you for who you are-when you finally find that person who sees perfection in your imperfections, acknowledge and appreciate them. Don't lose the moon while counting the stars- don't take their love for granted. Never think that they will stick around no matter how bad you treat them- instead, know that at a point in time, we all get tired waiting and move on. Don't lose that good woman or man to your ego, selfishness, unwillingness to accept that you have flaws, unnecessary nags, and etc. We all know a good man or woman when we find one but mostly we think that there are a lot of fishes in the sea and this results in us playing around them-wait till you lose the golden fish to realize you never had a lot of options but an illusion. The basis of every relationship should be love. Below are some key principles to a successful relationship.

MATURITY

It takes two matured beings to be in a relationship-if you are not ready to do away with your childish traits then relationship is definitely not your thing. Matters of the heart are never child's play-if you are not ready to quit sucking breasts to chew bones, please don't go in there to put another in pain. It takes a matured person to overlook certain things and guide us to become the very best of ourselves. Know that, no one can ever change another in a relationship-it only takes a matured person to compromise on a lot of things. Don't be a cry baby, accept your flaws when you go wrong and only work at making yourself a better person. Please, if you are not matured enough to nurse a heart, stay out! Lauren Martin once said that mature couples don't "fall in love", they step into it. Love isn't something you fall for; it's something you rise for.

Falling denotes lowering oneself, dropping down and being stuck somewhere lower than where you started. You have to get up from falling. Love isn't like that- at least not with people who are doing it right because love is either a passing game or forever. How can you tell if your relationship is in it for the long haul or the two-month plummet everyone predicted behind your love-obsessed back? First, it should be easy from the beginning to the end. Make sure there are no passionate fights with passionate make-up sex, there's no obsessive calling, texting or worrying, there's no real drama because drama is for kids. Drama is for people who don't know how to have a relationship-who live by idealistic, preconceived notions that love must be wild and obsessive. Love is easy. It is the easiest thing you've ever done. It's the calmest place in your life, the safest blanket you've ever worn. It is something that happens naturally; it doesn't need to be fought for day in and day out. You don't force your way into people's lives. That is not to say that there are no fights or arguments in love, there are but how you handle such shows your maturity.

Immature relationships are all about doubts. Does he love me? Is he cheating on me? Will we be together in two months? Mature couples don't need to ask questions. They already know the answers and they don't need reassurance from their partners. They are comfortable and secure and free of doubt because matured love isn't about all those questions but a comfort in knowing the big one is answered. If you constantly need a reassurance from your partner of his or her love, then I think it is better you quit since you don't know what you are into.

There's always a void in immature relationships. There is an apparent absence and incessant worry that something is missing. It burns you dimly even when together because there is a big vacuum of absence even in their presence. Matured people leave no voids because they know that they might be losing you to whatever that may be filling that void. They talk about issues when they feel they are gradually drifting apart and find ways to spice up their relationships.

Are you really matured to start a relationship?

RESPECT

Respect is key in every relationship- first of all is self-respect. Self-respect is like a magnetic force that draws respect from your partner to you. You don't expect to be respected when you in the first place do not respect yourself. Don't also forget that respect is reciprocal and thus you get what you give. If there is no respect between you too, then you might as well quit. Know when to move out and when to stay-don't create a room for disrespect from your partner all because you in the first place have failed to respect yourself. If you throw yourself at him, you will be used and dumped in the laundry basket because that's where dirty clothes end. Iron yourself out, have some self-respect, have an aim, don't try to pin him down with sex and above all, respect him.

Love without respect is dangerous-love is an essential key in every relationship. To respect is to understand that the other person is not you, not an extension of you, not a reflection of you, not your toy, not your pet, not your product. In a relationship of respect, your task is to understand that the other person is unique and learn how to mesh your needs with his or hers and help that person achieve what he or she wants to achieve. Your task is not to control the other person or try to change him or her in a direction that you desire.

Within every relationship, feeling anger, resentment, hurt or sadness is a natural occurrence. However, no matter the emotion you feel, respect should always be at the centre of the relationship. Your partner deserves to hear about your feelings in a way that is appropriate and feels respectful. Don't just walk out of a relationship without an explanation-no matter how angry you are, don't drop the call on them. Do unto others what you would have them do unto you. Respect!

44

EFFECTIVE COMMUNICATION

Effective Communication is an essential tool in every successful relationship. Communication allows us to interact with others, convey ideas, influence and etc. a relationship without an effective communication is a dead one. If you don't constantly speak to her to know her fears, pain, joy, successes and etc., someone else will and you should know constant communication between people increases the intimacy between them. Don't cry when you lose her to that person who gave her his time. A valuable time spent with your partner is never one at your free time but one that you made sacrifices to have. Many studies have identified that poor communication mostly wreck marriages and relationships. Good communication is never to be assumed; it requires practice. There is no magic pill to learn how to have effective conversations-you must learn how to express what you think constructively and without aggression or lack of respect, learn how to listen carefully. Listening builds trust, connection and intimacy.

In the midst of an argument, it's often hard to admit to having done something wrong or being the first to say `I'm sorry'. This is because there is a fear associated with it and defensiveness becomes a mechanism to defeat the fear. With practiced mindfulness, you will become increasingly skilled at identifying vulnerabilities. The more you are willing to be vulnerable first, the more likely it is for an argument to de-escalate. The fact that you accept the blame and say sorry doesn't always mean you are the one at fault- it only means that you are matured enough to tell the difference between peace and troubles.

Communication is an opportunity to grow closer to your partner. Once you master the tools of communication, you can discuss even the most sensitive of topics and still feel close and connected. This connection will strengthen your commitment and trust.

FAIRNESS

He who seeks equity must come with clean hands-don't expect what you are not willing to give. Some people are very selfish in their relationships- while we expect our partners to do something for us, we do otherwise. Some partners go to the extent of asking their partners to stay away from the opposite sex while they rather surround themselves with the opposite sex. Others will want to scroll through the phones of their partners but never will they want their phones to be touched. Others will want to force something on their partners but never willing to do same when asked of them. He who seeks equity must come with clean hands. Fairness must rule in every relationship- do unto your partner what you will want them to do to you.

We must not force on our partners what we want them to do- who says our ways are always right? Instead of commanding, ordering or instructing your partner, the goal should be to shift your focus on collaborating. Ask for your partner's opinion; include them in your thoughts and ideas so that you can be co-creators in your goals and life.

BE YOURSELF

You lose yourself when you try living for others-you fail to discover your true self when you get busy living a double life. You must be yourself in every relationship. Don't strive too hard to please your partner-if your partner loves you, he should be able to accept you for who you are. Be real to your partner- don't live a fake or double life to please. Let them know who you are and accept you for who you are. That way, you be at peace with yourself.

TRUST

Trust is the bedrock of every relationship. You can never love without trust, period! You don't start a relationship before looking for trust- how do you decide to be with someone you don't trust? We first trust before we surrender- as time goes on build the trust, trust like love grows. You start a foundation before building a house on it and that's how a relationship should also be. Trust is the foundation of every relationship. Without trust, there will always be doubts and problems in your relationship. If you can't trust your partner, just don't start a relationship with them because it will come crushing down. It is therefore advisable to know someone for a while before jumping into relationships with them, that way; you know whom you are dealing with-most will say that the best person to have a relationship with is your friend because they know you inside out and you know them too.

There are several keys to building a successful relationship aside these, which include spending quality time with your partner, appreciating them and recognizing their efforts, occasional gift surprises, telling them how much you love them, not taking them for granted, and not reducing the show of love only to the confines of the bedroom-let others know how you adore them amongst others.

MY TEN GOLDEN CODES FOR A BETTER RELATIONSHIP

1. No one can love you more than you love yourself

2. It is your sole duty to feel happy and free

3. Keep your partner closer and keep your family and friends close

4. Believe in the law of reciprocity; you get what you give

5. Everything has a lifespan but commitment and good management increases life span

6. No one is immune to pain

7. No one has the license to hurt another

8. Love alone is not enough

9. Walk out when you have to

10. Don't over-heighten your expectations ; anything can happen so like a soldier and a guide, always be prepared.

SEX.

Sex is part of our everyday life and we can't discuss life issues without talking about sex. Most people are of the assertion that sex strengthens the bond between couples though it is not always so, because for some, sex rather drifts them apart due to selfishness on the part of the other partner. It is mostly so hard for women to discuss their sexual preferences and issues with their partners because to most, it is a man's job but hey, sex is a mutual activity and no one's job. You have to contribute if you want to enjoy it- how do you expect your partner to know that you are not sexually satisfied when you have voiced nothing out? Research shows that about 8 out of 10 women have never had orgasm during sex with their partners but they might have had orgasm through masturbation. Yes, it is true that most men are selfish in bed and all they care about is jumping on you, entering and ejaculating but have you made an effort to take charge of the bedroom? Have you made an effort to let him know which part of your body gets aroused easily by the mildest touch? Have you told him that the clitoris is the most sensitive and the best place to touch to arouse a woman? Have you told him the sex position that gives you orgasm? Instead of lying all lazy in bed waiting for him to just jump on and off of you and complaining later that he's not good in bed, take charge! Sex is mutual!

A great sex life in a relationship strengthens the relationship and mostly keeps him from looking elsewhere for sex. Contribute to sexual decisions to be able to enjoy your sex life. Men must also learn more about the sexuality of women to be able to know the right things to do to please their partners- don't make her look elsewhere for sexual satisfaction, be the best you can be. A healthy sex life helps nurture love and intimacy in a relationship.

NATURAL APHRODISIACS FOR YOUR FEMALE LIBIDO

Lowered libido happens from time to time. The best advice is for women who experience diminished sex drive to slow down, take time to meditate and rest, get regular exercise and improve nutrition by eating a diet rich in plant-based whole foods. Natural supplements are safer for a libido boost. Aphrodisiacs are defined as foods, drinks or drugs that stimulate sexual desire. Below are some natural aphrodisiacs that can boost your libido;

1. Fenugreek; it has been used for centuries to boost female libido or stimulate sexual desires. It is used by both men and women to increase sex drive- it also promotes a healthy breast tissue and improves milk production in lactating mothers.it contains phytoestrogens and some say that it can increase breast size.

2. Warming spices; cinnamon, ginger and nutmeg are warming herbs that increase blood flow in the abdominal and pelvic regions. They are said to stimulate your appetite for both food and sex.

The blood-pumping effects of these delicious spices increase vaginal moisture and intensify sexual pleasure.

3. Ginseng; it is one of the best-selling natural aphrodisiacs for women. Ginseng triggers certain biochemical mechanisms in our body that increase libido.

4. Arginine; it is an amino acid that works as an aphrodisiac for women. Foods like nuts, cheese, eggs, meat etc. are rich in arginine. Arginine is responsible for the synthesis of nitric oxide which increases blood flow to the genitals. Arginine reduces vaginal dryness and stimulates orgasm in females. If it is taken with other supplements, it helps in clitoral sensation.

5. Chocolate; it helps to release serotonin, the feel-good chemical that helps to set the mood and stimulates sexual desire.

THE G-SPOT

The G-Spot or Grafenberg spot, named after the gynaecologist who first identified it is a mound of super-sensitive sponge like tissue located within the roof of the vagina, just inside the entrance. Proper stimulation of the G-spot can produce intense orgasms- because of its difficult-to-reach location and the fact that it is most successfully stimulated manually; the G-spot is not routinely activated for most women during vaginal intercourse. You must be sexually aroused to be able to locate your G-spot. To find it, try rubbing your finger in a beckoning motion along the roof of the vagina while you are in a squatting or sitting position or have your partner massage the upper surface of your vagina until you notice a particularly sensitive area. Some women tend to be more sensitive and can find the spot easily but for others, it's difficult.

During intercourse, many women feel that G-spot can be easily stimulated when the man enters from behind and when the woman is on top. Oral stimulation of the clitoris combined with manual stimulation of the G-spot can give a woman a highly intense orgasm.

HIGHTENING THE WOMAN'S SEXUAL DESIRE

Sexual desire disorder in women is in fact an extremely common condition. Women reporting low sexual desire also report low levels of arousal and sexual excitement and infrequent- of what use is it to have frequent sex when your partner cannot help you reach an orgasm. This all adds up to a lot of women feeling sexually dissatisfied- is it that the men are too selfish in the bedroom or they don't know the game of fore-play and how it prepares the woman mentally, physically and emotionally for sex? Women give many reasons for engaging in sex; for instance, the desire for emotional closeness, to please one's partner, to communicate intimately- all independent of a purely biological drive. In contrast to that of men who mostly do not consider so many reasons before having sex.

A woman with low sexual desire can feel shame and feelings of inadequacy. Conflict can be ignited between partners as the result of infrequent sex and lack of female initiation- most men complain that they are always the ones initiating and this can be laborious without considering the sexual physiology and psychology of women. Research shows that women do not experience strong sexual desire independent of environmental and relational clues- they will not initiate based on inner biological drive but will respond to a set of circumstances that are associated with romance, pleasure and intimacy. This fact calls for better attention in the sexual dance to "fore-fore play", the relationship dynamics, lowering stress levels and increasing romance in order to generate the "heat" if you will. Ignite the fire in her. According to Rosemary Basson and Dan Pollets, there are several factors which are relevant to female sexual desire and with reference to some of their works, they include;

1.Emotional Intimacy; the overall sense of emotional closeness, capacity to trust, and ability to communicate and be validated in this communication is highly related to a woman's availability and openness to become sexual. The adage that men seek out sex in order to feel close while women must feel close in order to become sexual might have some truth in it. It is therefore impossible to accurately assess low sexual desire in a woman without attending to the quality of relationship and level of emotional intimacy. The delight in an exquisite dining experience takes into consideration the setting, the service, the presentation of the food (appearance) as well as the actual taste. It also helps the overall enjoyment of the evening to find your dinning partner attractive and a good conversationalist. So men, ramp up your romance and seduction skills and you might ignite more "fire'.

2. Mental Health; the less a woman struggles with issues such as low self-esteem, poor body image, depression, anxiety and history of sexual/ physical/ emotional abuse, the greater the possibility that sex will be sought and enjoyed. Depression is strongly associated with reduced sexual function. Unfortunately and ironically, anti-depressants prescribed to treat depression especially SSRIs (Zoloft, Prozac, Paxil, etc.) typically have side effects which reduce sexual desire and arousal. In terms of sexual history, women who have a history where they were abused sexually or physically will retain aspects of the negative conditioning and can associate danger and threat with sexual intimacy. The messages that one absorbed about sexuality in the family of origin or religious training can also impact on adult sexuality. Growing up in a house that is hyper-religious and extremely repressive where for example, masturbation is deemed sinful, will lead to certain conclusions about sexuality. Clearly, overall mental health must be looked at in the assessment of female sexual desire disorder.

3. Sexual Context; this factor refers to how the sexual activity is experienced. This can include the feeling that her partner is being seductive and romantic, how much time is being taken in foreplay to assure arousal, and the skill level. In other words, how smooth and coordinated is the

sexual dance between you two. An important consideration is the sexual communication between you so that the need for necessary stimulation to augment arousal is signalled and responded to either verbally or non-verbally (non-verbal might be more graceful). This aids arousal and increases pleasure. Obviously, if the sexual experience is highly pleasurable, there will be future positive anticipation (expectation of reinforcement). A basic law of learning is that any behaviour that is highly reinforced has a greater probability of occurring in the future. If there is selfishness or lack of mutual satisfaction due to poor communication interplay between partners, sex will become at the very least unsatisfactory and obligatory.

4. Obstacles to mindful sex; another popular adage says that men are `unitaskers' and women are `multitaskers'. Men have an easier time focusing on the `hunt' and can block out distracting stimuli but women on the other hand are evolutionary wired to mind the home, kids, food, and community and are juggling many roles. Their awareness is often focused on many simultaneous demands. Perceived stress correlate poorly with a woman's availability to be sexual. Bassoon (2006) makes the point that women might go along with the sexual demand of her partner and not take responsibility for her own enjoyment and then come to expect a poor outcome or low satisfaction of her sexual relating. This of course leads to avoidance or sex being a low priority. Encouraging couples to discuss a more equitable sharing of domestic tasks and child care responsibility also makes sense in order to reduce the burden and lower stress levels.

5. Biological Factors; physical or biological factors can of course influence sexual desire and arousal. Depression was earlier mentioned-other factors that could affect sexual drive include diabetes, neurological disorders, vascular disease, high blood pressure and renal failure, diseases in the ovaries and/or low levels of androgen production can result in low desire and poor arousal.

YOUR AGE DOESN'T STOP YOU FROM ENJOYING YOUR SEX LIFE-TO THE MARRIED WOMEN, IGNITE THE FIRE TO KEEP YOUR HUSBANDS AT HOME.

PART TWO-

SOCIETAL CAVE

CHAPTER ONE

THE MISGUIDED AFRICAN PERCEPTION OF WOMEN.

Society has a far-reaching effect on people by shaping their belief systems, behaviours and values. Society and culture are inextricably linked, which affects an individual's taste in art, music and fashion and etc.-the society has influence on our being. An example is;

A child who grows up in a racist society is most likely to grow up as a racist and etc. it is an undeniable fact that in most parts of the world and not just Africa, women are treated as inferior beings but there has being a lot of bad judgments about the African perception of womanhood. Most have been misconstrued and escalated out of proportion. On the contrary to what the western world have portrayed the African perception of women to be as weak and etc., the African man holds in high esteem and cherishes the African woman and sees her as powerful and a good multi-tasked manager and that is why they entrust their homes to them. One who knows her history is a lost soul- never think that women abuse and the inferior perception of some men and societies is just African because it is a worldwide menace and on the contrary, African men revere and honour their women more than the others. Don't be fooled by someone's quest to run the whole African race down that the African woman is seen as feeble and mistreated and inferior. That is not to say that some men don't have a negative perception about women but please! This is not African- one's decision to run down another has got nothing to do with race but one's own fear of the strength and power the other gender carries.

Most men are naturally intimidated by intelligent and ambitious women and this again is NOT AFRICAN! Let's stop urging other races to run down our race because right from Adam, the African man has seen the African woman as a strong capable person and so don't relate someone's sick perception of African women being maids, weak and etc. to the entire race. It is their individual sickness not an entire race's- let's quit enjoying the jolly ride of being run down by other races. Ask yourself this, ARE THEY ANY BETTER? Let's go a little back into history; during the Black Rights Movements, the women empowered and strengthened the men on to fight their white masters who were oppressing them- the black woman was so powerful and behind all the decisions the black men were taking. The white men felt threatened by the power of the black woman and decided to cause a rift between the black man and the black woman - together we stand, divided we fall.

Thomas Babington Macaulay PC (Privy Council of the United Kingdom) popularly called, Lord Macaulay, was a British historian and a Whig Politician. In his view, Lord Macaulay divided the world into civilized nation and barbarism, with Britain representing the high point of civilization- yea, the same civilized nation who colonized, tortured, mistreated, raped our women and robbed Africans of a lot. Lord Macaulay, after visiting Africa for the first time is alleged to have reported back to Britain in these words in his address to the British Parliament on 2nd February, 1835;

"I have traveled across the length and breadth of Africa and I have not seen one person who is a beggar, who is a thief such wealth I have seen in this country, such high moral values, people of such caliber, that I do not think we would ever conquer this country unless we break the very backbone of this nation, which is her spiritual and cultural heritage and therefore, I propose that we replace her old and ancient education system, her culture, for if the Africans think that all that is foreign and English is good and greater than our own, they will lose their self-esteem, their native culture and they will become what we want them, a truly dominated nation",

Today, some parents nurture kids without even teaching them their native language-they even beat them up when they speak them. I know of a mother who beats up her son whenever he speaks Twi, which is her native language. You should be feeling ashamed of yourself for denying your child the right to know who they truly are. A nation without a history is a lost and vulnerable one- let's rise in unity and take over like the days of our fore-fathers. Today, we marry twice before we can call it marriage because after our traditional marriage, we do a "white wedding" which is the British traditional marriage and as ignorant as some pastors and Christians are, we have brought this into the church to the extent that, if one does not do a white wedding in the church, she is not considered married and is denied the right to certain privileges in the church including the taking of communion and occupying some church positions. We as "so called pastors" and "Christians" should be ashamed of ourselves for bringing into the church someone's traditional marriage and abandoning our own. Where in the Bible is that "church wedding?" Colonialism has gradually found its way into the church and it is pitiful. There is nothing like church wedding or white wedding in the Bible- it is someone's traditional marriage, let's respect our own. Marriage is just that union between the two families done at our traditional and true marriages.

The black community was growing so fast with the support of the women and family was and is still the strongest bond between blacks and again white supremacists were getting scared that the drive in the family will result in the blacks taking over and so they decided to break apart the family system of the blacks under the disguise of "Gender equality" and segregation and this collapsed our strong family ties of the extended family system where everyone looked out for each other to the selfish nuclear family system where no one cares about the third party. Have you asked yourself how many more successful person you would have had in your family if that your rich uncle had supported them? Have you asked yourself the reason why most people are depressed and emotionally tortured resulting in suicides and etc. all because we no longer care about the next person due to segregation? Do you realize that the African family system is the strongest and a prerequisite to move high the African? Do you realize you are only helping these other races break up your strength as a people so you fall? I am a family person so people of diverse opinions should bear with me- I love the old family homes, the rounded family homes in northern Ghana and etc. Do you know that many technology and inventions of the world were done by Africans but have lost it to others because we have failed to recognize our potential as a people? Today, Hippocrates is hailed as the modern father of medicine meanwhile Medicine and etc. started in Africa precisely Egypt with Imhotep? How much more of yourself do you want to lose? Hey! You are a strong race and most races out there feel threatened by your power and so, they always do things that will end up segregating you.

Nothing in this world is equal not even a set of Siamese twins- our biological make up and physiological make up alone distinguishes us from each other. We are two unique sexes that complement each other- we can never be equal! Why should you strive to be equal when you can stand out! Who told you that during those days, black women were not business owners, successful career women, and who told you that black husbands were not helping their wives with farm work, household chores and etc.? Have you asked yourself if you really understand the whole concept of gender equality? Who told you that you need to own a penis to make wealth, to be successful, to be good at what you do. Holy crap! We are solely entitled to our individual choices and career paths- no man is stopping you from being what you want to be. The only person who can stop you is yourself. Where were you when black women were making history in NASA? It was their individual choices to succeed and make history and not because they were fighting to own a penis. Oh yes, they faced adversities from people including women and men but their quest to stand out was greater than the adversities. A WOMAN CAN NEVER BE A MAN! And A MAN CAN NEVER BE A WOMAN! We are two different sexes- we complement each other- we are two incomplete halves who come together as one. Research shows that due to our distinct make-up, women are inclined to reading arts whereas men are more inclined to mathematics-this doesn't make anyone better than the other, we all meet halfway and make a perfect set.

Has any African man stopped you from making the good grades and pursing the courses you want? Why blame your lazy ass on an innocent race-are you not more concerned about appealing to a man sexually instead of intellectually? Has any man stopped you from occupying a higher position? Are there not great women out there doing great things? Did they need a penis to do that? Are there not men out there who help their wives and families with household chores? Are there not men out there who support their women to move up? Don't blame your laziness to move out of your comfort zone to explore and achieve on an entire race. Our lives are run by our individual choices not our gender! You reach for higher heights because you want to not because you are a woman or a man! Instead of sitting there and complaining, get up and work extra hard! Hard work and excellence and success know not gender! For God sake, stop the blame games. As I said earlier, it is an undeniable fact that some societies limit the opportunities given to women as compared to men but this is not AFRICAN! It is true that there are opportunistic men out there who take advantage of the fact that a woman needs a favour, position, work, help and etc to ask for sex in exchange of these but so are there some opportunistic women out there who do these though the men outnumber the women but this shouldn't stop you- there are so many ways to go around things. I remember when I had to forego a leadership ambition because I met so many of these opportunistic men- I was sad about this but I was equally happy that I didn't have to sell my body for a short term goal. I consoled myself with the fact that I don't need to hold a leadership position to be able to lead and cause a positive change- I could equally lead and cause a positive change without necessarily holding a leadership title and yea, I am. I didn't get discouraged by these opportunistic men but instead, I went around it in a different way. Let's tackle issues solely in relation to a particular individual or society and not a race. Are we not acting more racists to ourselves? In the African society, the woman rules the house and the man is just the face of the house- it is like saying that the man is the ceremonial head. What is more powerful than this? It seems the African woman is rather degrading herself and lowering herself to the ground without anyone forcing her there. ACCEPT THE POWER THAT YOU HAVE! YOU RULE!

Whoever said that the race you join to condemn your race is perfect? How can you follow the lecture of one who invades a black man's land, rapes women and children and even kill them. They forcibly took away black women away as slaves, wives and raped them- so you think this is an act of respect and a measure for judgment and comparison? You think these people who couldn't give equal opportunities to blacks and most especially black women should cut the rod for the measurement that treats the African fairly? I will recommend that you all watch the movie, HIDDEN FIGURES just so you know how three great black women suffered to make history. Let's attack individuals as the monsters they are, let's attack fathers who limit the opportunities available for their girl child, let's attack that husband that mistreats his wife, let's attack the society that dehumanizes the woman, let's attack the religious leader who relegate women to the ground as the individuals that they are rather than attacking a whole race because on the contrary, the African family system is the strongest ever and the African man cherishes and loves his woman. I don't have the right to call all African women irresponsible all because I had a tough time with my mum growing up-hell no!

WOMAN ACTIVISM AND FEMINISM.

According to Saumya Dubey, Feminism is the advocacy of women's rights on the ground of the sexes thus all feminist movements share a common goal: to establish and achieve political, economic, personal and social rights for women that are equal to those of men. Before I continue may I ask you this; which law in Ghana states that women shouldn't occupy positions or be in parliament or take up leadership positions? Which law asks that no woman is taken to school? There is none right? So get this straight, these movements are not there to fight men to put you in a position- they can fight all they want but if you as a person is not ready to improve on yourself, aim higher and have ambitions which you work hard to achieve, they will be fighting in vain. Besides, they are not there to fight men but to orient you well and heighten your libido for success so that as an individual, you see the need to rise above your circumstances to achieve the best.

Lately, the word has caught a lot of wrong fire. People have started treating feminism to be synonymous with asking women to be `masculine', to be man-hating- these are all the things feminism wasn't ever about. In fact, feminism doesn't ask you to treat a woman special, it's the exact opposite- to treat her no different from a man. It is to let her have equal rights-human rights. Feminism is never about begging men to give us a quota in parliament or leadership positions- it's about working hard to achieve that with our capabilities not our pitiful faces. It is the quest for an equal platform so that you won't plead with electorates to vote for you because you are a woman but because you are more capable than your male contender- this is true feminism.

Being a feminist means liberating and empowering women to take control of their life choices- to be a housewife or a single working mom, to be a fashion designer or a politician, to wear a bikini or `jalabia'- let her decide.

CHAPTER TWO

THE TRUE AFRICAN SOCIETAL PERCEPTION OF WOMANHOOD.

There is no difference in gender; every woman is a true woman no matter the race. I am only making this race factor inclusive because most people of the other races have taken it upon themselves to run down the black race including calling Black women lazy which I strongly beg to differ. If there is any race that portrays the strength of women, it is the African. From the home to work throughout our every stage of life, the strong African woman exists. I am not a racist and so I have no time to run down another race- the truth is, you only run down someone who is better than you and can never be. I am a proud African woman and I need no race to dispute that. I only write this to let the whole world know the True African Perception of womanhood and rubbish the nonsense perception out there. The African race holds and cherishes women.

The feminization of most significant elements like the earth as in "Asaase Yaa" meaning, "mother earth", events in history, countries and our current times is not accidental. Women are so powerful that, they can make and unmake men. In the African setting, that powerful trait in women is shown when Queens rather can make and unmake kings. This shows how the African race holds the woman in high esteem contrary to the assertions of some racists that the African man mistreats his woman. In most of the African culture, chiefs are enstooled or enskinned by Queens and they also have the power to destool them when they violate the laws of the land. This power is vested in the African woman because, the African woman is seen as one who though human and can be fallible is close to perfection and makes right and sound judgements which is why she is entrusted with the power to make and unmake the rulers of the people- if she objects to anyone's candidature, it ends there because she is seen as an epitome of sound judgement and wisdom. The African holds in high esteem their women, which is why women are powerful.

African women deserve eternal glorification and the accolade for the strongest women on earth and African men acknowledge the nature-given power of women, given that they manage to wield together perfectly a livelihood for their families, raise children, keep the family bond alive, and withstand the relentless matrimonial demands from some irresponsible husbands amid an overwhelming insufficiency of resources. African women are the most supportive of all- while elsewhere, a husband is under pressure to maintain the flow of resources and must even loan money from his wife to be able to cater for the very family of which his very wife is part, the African woman acts very supportive even in hard times. To keep her family together, she can go to the length of even hiding the fact that her husband is financially down and take over the management of the household without even letting her children in on the situation- this is just to keep the respect that exists between father and children at home. The African man acknowledges all these and respects the African woman for the pillar she is. A friend of mine told me a story of how he only grew up to find out that it was her mother who had been paying her fees and taking care of every other thing at home -her mother had hidden the fact that her husband's job had collapsed and continually told her kids that, "daddy says use this for your fees... or that". The African woman is the pillar of the African man that which he acknowledges.

The African woman is focused and strong and that is why she can multi-task. That is why she is able to juggle between managing her home, raising kids, managing her man, managing her job, managing family, handling pressures of work, family and etc. and she does all perfectly- is the African woman not a super woman to be able to do all these? It takes one who is physically, emotionally and mentally strong and focused to be able to juggle between all these. The African society acknowledges this strength and focus and that is why it is able to entrust all these into the hands of the woman. How many men can juggle between these?-they already are even tired from their uni-tasking. The black woman has been strong and focused right from colonization through to the independence of Africa to now- our strength has never died. While some of the westerners left their wives home to sew and knead, the black woman stood in the front line and fought for their husbands and to keep their families intact because the family bond has always been the strength of Africa.

Before the whites came to Africa, African women were held in high esteem by their men and still are, they were opinion leaders, they made kings and they were and still are the power and strength of the African family. There may have been some black men who were mistreating their wives and so were there some white men doing same but this is individual traits and a whole race cannot be run down because of another man's weakness. The African family bond was the greatest and strongest and still is- most of the Whites envied. On the other hand, most of these Whites left their wives home to sew, make babies and cook. They came here to rape our women and have the guts to preach division and point fingers at the Black man who protects his woman as one who mistreats them to break our families apart. They claim African women have been reduced to slaves when they rather made slaves out of their women and captured the Black women as slaves. How can a drunkard be advising the sane? I am not a racist but I am a proud African woman and I advocate for the right history to be written. Enough of the lies! We will write our own stories. Enough of the history and identity stealing, Africa shall rise!

Did they treat us any better? Female slaves were given brutal and degrading forms of punishment. Slaves were punished by whipping, shackling, beating, mutilation, branding and/or imprisonment. Pregnancy was never a barrier to a female slave getting punished. Slave masters would dig a hole big enough for the woman's stomach to lie in and proceed with lashings. Angela Davis contends that the systematic rape of female slaves is analogous to the medieval concept of "droit du seigneur" believing that rape was a deliberate effort by slave masters to extinguish resistance in women and reduce them to the status of animals. Children of slaves were subjected to sexual abuse by their masters, the masters' children and relatives. Even men were also sexually abused. In 1662, the southern colonies in the United States adopted into law the principle of "partus sequitur ventrem" by which the children of slave women took the status of their mothers. The law relieved their slave masters who raped and impregnated the female slaves of the responsibility to support their children. Don't you think that the African continent has undergone serious mental and psychological changes after the colonization? I told you earlier that most often than not, our past experiences and environment shape us; it is therefore not surprising that some individuals mistreat their women and some women also rebel against their men- going through such a torture is never easy and sometimes might have a lasting effect on them.

As Michelle Obama once said, "there are still many causes worth sacrificing for, so much history yet to be made"-we are too strong and have come a long way to be run down by another race. Let's keep rising and impacting- if just three black women at NASA, Katherine Johnson, Dorothy Vaughan and Mary Jackson could make a huge difference and just one strong brave Black woman, Nana Yaa Asantewaa, could lead a battalion of male warriors for the fight for justice, Dode Akaabi could start the culture of kings and queens sitting on stools and adorning themselves with golden ornaments which still lives today and Oprah Winfrey is still out there making a difference and showing our strength, what stops us all from rising and roaring. We are strong, we are bold, we are beautiful, we are brave, we are pace setters, and we are the PROUD AFRICAN WOMEN. Let us take inspiration from great black women like Rosa Parks who was a human rights activist who fought against segregation, Marjorie Joyner who was a beauty salon owner and changed the game of hair styling when she invented the "permanent wave machine" and a scalp protector, Mary Kenner, Ruane Jeter who invented the toaster, Alice Parker who designed a gas heating furnace, Mary McLeod Bethune, a pioneer for education and a civil rights activist, Ellen Johnson-Sirleaf who is the world's first Black female President and Africa's first female head of State, Coretta Scott King, wife of Dr. Martin Luther King and a civil and women's rights activist, Condoleeza Rice who was the first black woman to serve as the US National Security Adviser and Secretary of State and the first Black female to hold the position of Provost at Stanford University, Oprah Winfrey, Harriet Tubman who was a true warrior against slavery, Ella Baker who was a dedicated civil rights activist, Harriet McDaniel, who was the first Black woman to win an Oscar in 1940, Maya Angelou, a legendary poet and award-winning author, Ida B. Wells who was a renowned journalist, Shirley Chisholm who was the first Black Congresswoman and the first major-party black candidate to run for President of the United States, Sojourner Truth who was a true feminist who fought for women's rights and to abolish slavery, Diahann Carroll who was the first Black woman to star in her own television series and scored an Emmy and Golden Globe, Dame Eugenia Charles who was Caribbean's first female Prime Minister, Joyce Banda who was first female President of Malawi and many others.

Ghana can also boast of great women like, Nancy Abu- Bonsrah who is the first Black female to be matched at John Hopkins University of Medicine in the Department of Neurosurgery, Nana Konadu Agyemang Rawlings who is the first female candidate to contest the position of the flag bearer of the National Democratic Congress, Theodosia Okoh who designed the Ghana national flag and acknowledged as the godmother of Ghanaian Hockey, Alice Anum, the first real star of female athletics, whose original nickname "Baby Jet" has been inherited by current Black Stars captain, Asamoah Gyan, Mercy Tagoe who was in the Ghana National female football team, the Black Queens and now an accomplished referee assuming a role as one of Ghana's first female FIFA Referees, Adwoa Bayor who is arguably Ghana's greatest football player of all time, Senyuiedzorm Adadevoh who is one of Africa's most rated and most respected sports photographers and CEO of the "Firm Images Image", and others.

These women are just a handful of the many that have made and continue to make a huge difference to the world. What stops you from achieving greater heights? If they could and still do, what then is our reason to sit back, relax and fail?

CHAPTER THREE

SOME GREAT AFRICAN WOMEN WHO LIVED.

So many great African women lived and made history and I already mentioned some in the previous chapter. I would like to mention and discuss a few more in this chapter.

DODE AKAABI

I am the great grand-daughter of this great woman but I write this purposely to preserve history devoid of any emotional sentiments and personal association with the character and I do this reference to Archives of the history of the Obutus , History of the Gas, mijaku.com, http://gadangmenikasemoasafo.wordpress.com, www.ghanaculture.gov.gh/index1, Kwame Ampene, founder of the Guan historical society and writer of the history of the Awutus, oral tradition from some elders and http://muse.jhu/edu.

Dode Akaabi, the grand-daughter of Wettey, the leader of the Obutus (Awutus), one of the Guan tribes and a princess of Obutu married one of the king of the Gas, Mampon Okai also known as Dua Kwei and bore him a son by name, Okaikwei. Dode means ancient. The Obutus (Awutus) established a good relationship with the Gas who before their encounter with the Obutus had their "Wulomos" (spiritual leaders) leading them. The Obutus had kings and the association of the Gas with them led to their commencement of kings ruling instead of the Wulomos. Till now, though the Awutus are Guans, they are also considered as Gas by others because of Dode Akaabi's rule in the Ga land and the miscegenation between the Gas and the Obutus (Awutus). The Awutus and Senya Bereku was assimilated into the family of Naiwe in the Ga land and till date, the ruling families of Awutu and Senya Bereku bear the title of "Nai" in recognition of their blood relationships with the Gas. The Obutus (Awutus) also intermarried with the Akwamus and other tribes and so there are some historians that refer to the Akwamus as Guans. In 1693, the Asamani of Akwamu who is believed to be from the Asamani clan in the Obutu/Guan tribe led a raid and seized Osu Castle from the Danish colonists. There is also the 'Tutu' shrine in Bereku where it is believed that Manu Kotosii, the mother of Osei Tutu1went to seek help from the Tutu shrine for a son whom was named Osei Tutu1though the Akwamus have a different story.

Dode Akaabi, wife of the Ga Mantse then, Mampon Okai, also known as Dua Kwei and mother of Okaikwei ruled as the first female king of the Gas and Obutus after the demise of Mmpon Okai due to the fact that, the heir to the throne, Okaikwei, who was too young at the time of the demise of the king. Her rule was repugnant to the Ga customary law of succession which only allowed male rulers. She was the caretaker of the late king's regalia and paraphernalia and doubled as his wife. She emerges as a formidable figure whose rise as the first female political leader of the Gold Coast opened a new vistas of power to her gender. She is generally believed to have introduced much display of jewellery and colourful attire into the chieftains' institution. Some even attribute the custom of sitting on stools to her. Prior to her rule, stools were mainly taken to war and held aloft to lift the spirit of the troops. Since her authority, unlike her predecessors was no longer derived from privileged access to the deity, she had to formulate new methods of governance. This she did principally through the previous untried method of direct legislation which appears to have drawn the ire of her subjects. She brought a new magnificence to royalty by combining western culture with new standards of culture. She demanded to sit on the war stool to visually symbolize her authority over her people and this led to the beginning of kings and queens sitting on stools.

She forbade men from using the expression, `bulu' (fool) in reference to their wives and when they did; she ordered that a live lion or tiger be captured for her just to deter the men from disrespecting their wives. She led the Guans comprising the Obutus, Lartehs, Kyereponis, Krachis, and etc to secure so many lands which included Ayawaso, Nsakina, Ablekuma, Amasaman, etc and helped the Akwamus in so many wars. She had her personal war stools which present day are in Bereku and Larteh which she took to wars and trained most of the Akwamu warriors.

NANA YAA ASANTEWAA- COMMANDER-IN-CHIEF.

No woman is known in the history of the African reactions and responses to European power better than Nana Yaa Asantewaa , queen mother of Ejisu, an Asante state in the Ashanti region of Ghana. She was the military leader of the "Yaa Asantewaa War" or the " War of the Golden Stool" in 1900, which was the last war between the Asantes and the British and during which she became referred to by the British as the "Joan D'Arc of Africa". Her dream for an Asante free of British rule was realized on 6th March 1957, when the Asante protectorate gained independence as part of Ghana, the first African nation in the sub-Saharan Africa to achieve this feat. Great women like her started the war on colonization and she will never be forgotten- today, a statue in memory of her bravery and contributions stands at Ejisu.

MIRIAM MAKEBA

Another prominently outspoken and visible opponent of South Africa's apartheid regime was Miriam Makeba, also known as Mama Africa and the empress of African Music. Makeba was not only involved in radical activity against apartheid but also in the civil rights movement and then black power. She said, "Everybody now admits that apartheid was wrong and all I did was tell the people who wanted to know where I come from how we lived in South Africa. I just told the world the truth and if my truth then becomes political, I can't do anything about that".

NZINGHA

Nzingha, also known as Ann Nzingha, is the great national figure of pre-colonial Angola. The extraordinary scholar, John Henrik Clarke, referenced her as the "greatest military strategist that ever confronted the armed forces of Portugal." Nzingha was born in Central Africa around 1582 and her brilliance was recognised early on. The fact that she was a woman was not an impediment to her ability to lead. Toward the middle of her life, she became increasingly aggressive in her desire to maintain the power and dignity of the people of Central Africa. Indeed, her military campaigns kept the Portuguese in Africa at bay for more than four decades. Her goal was the final and complete eradication of the Portuguese capture and enslavement of African people. She sent ambassadors and representatives throughout West and Central African with the goal of building a massive coalition of Africans to eject the Portuguese.

MAKEDA

During the 10th century B.C. we hear of the deeds of Makeda- a near-legendary African woman. This queen had the qualities of an outstanding ruler and seems to have governed over a prosperous land encompassing parts of both East Africa and Southwest Asia. In the Quran, she is known as "Bilqis', in the great epic of Ethiopia called the "Kebra Negast", she is called Makeda and in the Bible and in the popular imagination of the western world, she is known as the Queen of Sheba. These texts show an unmistakable image of a well-developed land characterized by the elevated posture of women and Makeda was not an isolated phenomenon.

PART THREE

THE WOMAN AND HER HEALTH.

CHAPTER ONE

MENSTRUATION

Menstruation, also known as a period or monthly, is the monthly discharge of blood and mucosal tissue from the inner lining of the uterus through the vagina. The first period usually begins between twelve and fifteen years of age, a point in time known as menarche. However, periods may occasionally start as young as eight years old and still be considered normal. The average age of the first period is generally later in the developing world and earlier in the developed world. The typical length of time between the first day of one period and the first day of the next is 21 to 45 days in young women and 21 to 31 days in adults with an average of 28 days. Bleeding usually lasts around 2 to 7 days. Menstruation stops occurring after menopause, which usually occurs between 45 and 55 years of age. Periods also stop during pregnancy and typically do not resume during the initial months of breastfeeding. There have been insignificant number of cases where the woman still bleeds during the first trimester.

Up to 80% of women report having some symptoms prior to menstruation. Common signs and symptoms include acne, tender breasts, bloating, feeling tired, irritability, and mood changes. Menstruation in other animals occurs in primates, such as apes and monkeys as well as bats and the elephant shrew.

The menstrual cycle occurs due to the rise and fall of hormones. This cycle results in the thickening of the lining of the uterus and the growth of ovaries (eggs). The egg is released from an ovary around day fourteen in the cycle; the thickening lining of the uterus provides nutrients to an embryo after implantation. If pregnancy does not occur, the lining is released in what is known as menstruation. Perimenopause is when fertility in a female declines and menstruation occurs less regularly in the years leading up to the final menstrual period, when a female stops menstruating completely and is no longer fertile.

AMENORRHEA

Amenorrhea is the absence of menstrual periods in a woman during her reproductive years. Amenorrhoea is classified as either `primary' (menstrual periods not having started by age 16 years) or `secondary' which is the absence of menstrual periods in a woman who has previously been menstruating for six months or more. It is important to remember that amenorrhea is normal before puberty, during pregnancy and after the menopause. Women may also experience amenorrhoea while breastfeeding (lactation). It may be caused by the many factors including;

1.Defects in one or more areas of the reproductive system such as the hypothalamus and pituitary gland (parts of the brain regulating reproduction), ovaries, uterus or vagina.

2. A side-effect from treatment for cancer

3. A symptom of endometrial cancer.

One of the most common types of amenorrhea is `functional hypothalamic amenorrhea'. This is where the onset of amenorrhea can be linked to factors such as recent stress, change in weight, excessive dieting or exercise or illness.

Patients may have the following signs and symptoms of amenorrhea in addition to the absence of menstrual periods;

1.Headache, visual disturbance or tiredness caused by diseases affecting the pituitary gland

2. Spontaneous flow of milk from the breasts caused by excessive levels of a hormone called prolactin. This is called galactorrhoea

3. Acne and/or excess body hair growing in male pattern distribution caused by polycystic ovary syndrome

4. Symptoms of premature menopause (premature ovarian syndrome) such as hot flashes, vaginal dryness, poor sleep or reduced libido

5. Short stature and lack of secondary sexual characteristics (eg. Breast development) which is normally caused by the genetic condition, Turner syndrome

Treatment of amenorrhoea depends on the underlying cause. Women are counselled regarding the cause and management of amenorrhoea and their reproductive potential. A number of treatments are available including;

1.Women who are very underweight through not eating enough or exercising too much often do not have periods; this may be resolved by putting on weight and/or exercising less

2. Surgery and/or medication may be required for pituitary conditions. Women with tumours secreting excess prolactin are treated with a class of drugs called `dopamine agonists', which reduce prolactin levels

3. Hormone replacement therapy (oestrogen plus progesterone in those with an undamaged uterus)

4. Prescribing the missing hypothalamic or pituitary hormones that regulate reproduction for women who want to be pregnant.

5. Surgery may be required in patients with uterine or vaginal abnormalities dating from birth.

HEALTH EFFECTS OF MENSTRUATION

In most women, various physical changes are brought about by fluctuations in hormone levels during the menstrual cycle. This includes muscle contractions of the uterus (menstrual cramping) that can precede or accompany menstruation. Some may notice water retention, changes in sex drive, fatigue, breast tenderness, or nausea. Breast swelling and discomfort may be caused by water retention during menstruation. Usually, such sensations are mild and some females notice very few physical changes associated with menstruation. A healthy diet, reduced consumption of salt, caffeine and alcohol, and regular exercise may be effective for women in controlling some symptoms. Severe symptoms that disrupt daily activities and functioning may be diagnosed as premenstrual dysphoric disorder.

CRAMPS

Many women experience painful cramps, also known as dysmenorrhea, during menstruation. Pain results from ischemia and muscle contractions. Spiral arteries in the secretory endometrium constrict, resulting in ischemia to the secretory endometrium. This allows the uterine lining to slough off. The myometrium contracts spasmodically in order to push the menstrual fluid through the cervix and out of the vagina. The contractions are mediated by a release of prostaglandins.

Painful menstrual cramps that result from an excess of prostaglandin release are referred to as primary dysmenorrhea. Primary dysmenorrhea usually begins within a year or two of menarche, typically with the onset of ovulatory cycles. Treatments that target the mechanism of pain include Non-Steroidal Anti-Inflammatory Drugs (NSAIDs) and hormonal contraceptives. NSAIDs inhibit prostaglandin production. With long-term treatment, hormonal birth control reduces the amount of uterine fluid/ tissue expelled from the uterus thus resulting in shorter, less painful menstruation. These drugs are typically more effective than treatments that do not target the source of the pain (eg. Acetaminophen). For many women, primary dysmenorrhea gradually subsides in late second generation. Pregnancy has also been demonstrated to lessen the severity of dysmenorrhea, when pregnancy resumes. However, dysmenorrhea can continue until menopause; 5-15% of women with dysmenorrhea experience symptoms severe enough to interfere with daily activities.

Secondary dysmenorrhea is the diagnosis given when menstruation pain is a secondary cause to another disorder. Conditions causing secondary dysmenorrhea include endometriosis, uterine fibroids and uterine adenomyosis. Rarely, congenital malformations, Intra-Uterine Devices, certain cancers and pelvic infections can cause secondary dysmenorrhea. Symptoms include pain spreading to hips, lower back and thighs, nausea and frequent diarrhoea or constipation. If the pain occurs between menstrual periods, lasts longer than the first few days of the period or is not adequately relieved by the use of non-steroidal anti-inflammatory drugs or hormonal contraceptives, women should be evaluated for secondary causes of dysmenorrhea.

MOOD AND BEHAVIOUR

Some women experience emotional disturbances starting one or two weeks before their period and stopping soon after the period has started some even continue to have these emotional disturbances during the period. Symptoms may include mental tension, irritability, mood swings and crying spells. Problems with concentration and memory may occur. There may also be depression or anxiety.

BLEEDING

The average volume of menstrual fluid during a monthly menstrual period is 35 milliliters. Menstrual fluid is the correct name for the flow although many people prefer to refer to it as menstrual blood. Menstrual fluid contains some blood, as well as cervical mucus, vaginal secretions and endometrial tissue. Menstrual fluid is reddish-brown, a slightly darker colour than venous blood. The blood contains sodium, phosphate, iron, and chloride, the extent of which depends on the woman.

MENSTRUAL DISORDERS

There is a wide spectrum of differences in how women experience menstruation. There are several ways that someone's menstrual cycle can differ from the norm, any of which should be discussed with a doctor to identify the underlying cause: infrequent menstrual periods (oligomenorrhea), short or extremely light periods (hypomenorrhea), too frequent periods defined as more frequently than every 21 days (polymenorrhea), extremely heavy or long periods (hypermenorrhea), extremely painful periods (dysmenorrhea), breakthrough bleeding also called spotting (metrorrhagia) and absent periods (amenorrhea). Dysfunctional uterine bleeding is a hormonally caused bleeding abnormality. It typically occurs in pre-menopausal women who do not ovulate normally. All these bleeding abnormalities need medical attention; they may indicate hormone imbalances, uterine fibroids, or other problems.

Women who have undergone female genital mutilation may experience menstrual problems such as slow and painful menstruation that is caused by the near-complete sealing off of the vagina.

CHAPTER TWO

MENOPAUSE

Menopause literally means the `end of monthly cycles' from the Greek word, `pausis' which means pause and `men' which means month. Menopause, also known as the climacteric, is the time in most women's lives when menstrual periods stop permanently, and they are no longer able to bear children. Menopause typically occurs between 49 and 52 years of age. Medical professionals often define menopause as having occurred when a woman has not had any vaginal bleeding for a year. It may also be defined by a decrease in hormone production by the ovaries. In those who have had surgery to remove their uterus but they still have ovaries, menopause may be viewed to have occurred at the time of the surgery or when their hormone levels fell. Following the removal of the uterus, symptoms typically occur earlier, at an average of 45 years of age. Before menopause, a woman's periods typically become irregular; which means that periods may be longer or shorter in duration or be lighter or heavier in the amount of flow. During this time, women often experience hot flashes; typically last from 30 seconds to ten minutes and may be associated with shivering, sweating and reddening of the skin. Other symptoms may include vaginal dryness, trouble sleeping and mood changes. The severity of symptoms varies between women. While menopause is often thought to be linked to an increase in heart disease, this primarily occurs due to increasing age and does not have a direct relationship with menopause.

· Menopause is usually a natural change. It can occur earlier in those who smoke tobacco and other causes include surgery that removes both ovaries and some types of chemotherapy. At the psychological level, menopause happens because of a decrease in the ovaries' production of the hormone levels in the blood or urine.

DIAGNOSIS

One way of assessing the impact on women of some of these menopause effects are the Greene Climacteric Scale questionnaire, the Cervantes Scale and the menopause rating scale.

Pre-menopause is a term used to mean the years leading up to the last period; when the levels of reproductive hormones are becoming more variable and lower and the effects of hormone withdrawal are present. Pre-menopause starts same time before the monthly cycles become noticeably irregular in timing.

Perimenopause which literary means, `around the menopause', refers to the menopause transition years, a time before and after the date of the final episode of flow. According to the North American Menopause Society, this transition can last for four to eight years. The Centre for Menstrual Cycle and Ovulation Research describes it as a six to ten year phase ending 12 months after the last menstrual period. During Perimenopause, oestrogen levels average about 20-30% higher than during pre-menopause, often with wide fluctuations. These fluctuations cause many of the physical changes during Perimenopause as well as menopause. Some of these changes are hot flashes, night sweats, difficulty sleeping, vaginal dryness, or atrophy, incontinence, osteoporosis and heart disease. During this period, fertility diminishes but is not considered to reach zero until the official date of menopause. The official date is determined retroactively, once 12 months have passed after the last appearance of menstrual blood. The menopause transition typically begins between 40 and 50 years of age with average being 47. Some research appears to show that melatonin supplementation in Perimenopausal women can improve thyroid function and gonadotropin levels as well as restoring fertility and menstruation and preventing depression associated with menopause.

Post-menopausal describes women who have not experienced any menstrual flow for a minimum of 12 months, assuming they have a uterus and are not pregnant or lactating. In women without a uterus, post-menopause can be identified by a blood test showing a very high Follicle-Stimulating Hormone (FSH) level. Post-menopause is therefore the period in a woman's life when her ovaries become inactive. Any period-like flow during post-menopause, even spotting, must be reported to a doctor. The cause may be minor but the possibility of endometrial cancer must be checked for.

MANAGEMENT OF MENOPAUSE

Menopause is a natural stage of life. It is not a disease or a disorder. Therefore, it does not automatically require any kind of medical treatment. However, in those cases where the physical, mental and emotional effects are strong enough that they significantly disrupt the life of the woman experiencing them, palliative medical therapy may sometimes be appropriate. These are some of the ways by which menopause can be managed;

HORMONE REPLACEMENT THERAPY

In the context of the menopause, Hormone Replacement Therapy (HRT) is the use of oestrogen in women without a uterus and oestrogen plus progestin in women who have an intact uterus. HRT may be reasonable for the treatment of menopausal symptoms such as hot flashes and osteoporosis; however, its use appears to increase the risk of strokes and blood clots. When used for menopausal symptoms, it should be used for the shortest time possible and at the lowest dose possible. The response to HRT in each postmenopausal woman may not be the same. It appears effective for preventing bone loss and osteoporotic fracture. There is some concern that this treatment increases the risk of breast cancer. Adding testosterone to hormone therapy has a positive effect on sexual function of postmenopausal women, although it may be accompanied by hair growth, acne and a reduction in High-Density Lipoprotein (HDL) cholesterol. These side effects diverge depending on the doses and methods of using testosterone.

OTHER THERAPIES

1. Lack of lubrication is a common problem during and after Perimenopause. Vaginal moisturizers can help women with overall dryness and lubricants can help with lubrication difficulties that may be present during intercourse. It is worth pointing out that moisturizers and lubricants are different products for different issues: some women complain that their genitalia are uncomfortably dry all the time, and they may do better with moisturizers. Those who need only lubricants do well using them only during intercourse.

2. Low-dose prescription vaginal oestrogen products such as oestrogen creams are generally a safe way to use oestrogen topically, to help vaginal thinning and dryness problems while only minimally increasing the levels of oestrogen in the bloodstream.

3. In terms of managing hot flashes, lifestyle measures such as drinking cold liquids, staying in cool rooms, using fans, removing excess clothing and avoiding hot flash triggers such as hot drinks, spicy foods, etc. may partially supplement or even obviate the use of medications for some women.

4. Individual counselling or support groups can sometimes be helpful to handle sad, depressed, anxious, or confused feelings women may be having as they pass through what can be for some a very challenging transition time.

5. Osteoporosis can be minimized by smoking cessation, adequate Vitamin D intake and regular weight-bearing exercise. The Bisphosphate drug, Alendronate, may decrease the risk of a fracture.

CHAPTER THREE-

URINARY TRACT HEALTH

Women are very much exposed to getting Urinary Tract Infections or UTI and some experts rank a woman's lifetime risk of getting one as high as 1 in 2 with many women having repeat infections, sometimes for years unending. The urinary tract comprises the bladder, kidney, ureters and urethra. A UTI is an infection of any part of the Urinary system. Most infections involve the lower urinary tract. UTIs are given names depending on where they occur like Bladder infection which is Cystitis, Urethra infection which is Urethritis and kidney infection which is Pyelonephritis. The ureters are very rarely the site of infection. Women are more likely to develop UTIs than men due to anatomical differences; the urethra is shorter in women than in men and it is closer to the anus, making it more likely that bacteria are transferred to the bladder. Pregnant women are more likely to develop UTI than other women, if one does occur, it is likely to travel up to the kidneys; this is because of anatomical changes during pregnancy that affect the urinary tract. UTI in pregnant women can be very dangerous to both the mother and the foetus. Most pregnant women are tested for the presence of bacteria in their urine, even if there are no symptoms, and treated with antibiotics to prevent spread. It is therefore very advisable for pregnant women to visit the hospital for pre-natal care not doing away with ante-natal care too.

Most UTIs are not serious but can lead to serious problems, particularly with upper UTIs. Recurrent or long-lasting kidney infections (chronic) can cause permanent damage and some kidney infections (acute) can be life threatening, particularly if septicaemia (bacteria entering the bloodstream) occurs. They can also increase the risk of women delivering low birth weight or premature babies.

CAUSES OF UTIs

UTIs are a key reason we are often told to wipe from front to back after using the bathroom. That is because the urethra, the tube that transports urine from the bladder to the outside of the body, is located close to the anus. Bacteria from the large intestine such as Escherichia Coli (E. coli), are in the perfect position to escape the anus and invade the urethra. From there, they can travel up to the bladder and if the infection is not treated, continue to infect the kidneys. Sex can introduce bacteria to the urinary tract too especially having anal and vaginal sex at the same time-the penis can pick the E. coli from the anus and infect the urethra. The following factors can also increase the likelihood of developing a UTI;

- Sexual intercourse (especially if more frequent, intense and with multiple or new partners)
- Diabetes
- Poor personal hygiene
- Problems emptying the bladder completely
- Having a urinary catheter
- Bowel incontinence
- Blocked flow of urine
- Kidney stones
- Some forms of contraception
- Pregnancy
- Menopause
- Procedures involving the Urinary Tract
- Suppressed immune system
- Use of spermicides and tampons
- Heavy use of antibiotics (which can disrupt the natural flora of the bowel and urinary tract)

SYMPTOMS OF UTIs

The symptoms of UTI can depend on age, gender, the presence of a catheter and what part of the urinary tract has been infected. Common symptoms of UTI include;

- Strong and frequent urge to urinate
- Cloudy, bloody or strong smelling urine
- Pain or burning sensation when urinating
- Nausea and vomiting
- Muscle aches and abdominal pains
- Feeling tired or shaky
- Fever or chills (a sign that the infection may have reached your kidneys)

TESTS AND DIAGNOSIS

Diagnosis will usually be made after asking about the symptoms and testing a urine sample to assess the presence of white blood cells, red blood cells and bacteria. A method of collecting urine called `clean catch' is used, which is where a person washes their genital area before collecting a urine sample mid-flow. This helps to prevent bacteria from around the genital area getting caught in the sample. If a person has recurrent UTIs, a doctor may request further diagnostic testing to determine if anatomical issues or functional issues are to blame. Such tests may include;

Diagnostic imaging: assessing the urinary tract using ultrasound, CT and MRI scanning, radiation tracking or X-rays.

Urodynamics : a procedure that determines how well the urinary tract is storing and releasing urine.

Cystoscopy: looking inside the bladder and urethra with a camera lens inserted via the urethra through a long thin tube.

TREATMENT OF UTIs

As UTIs are normally caused by bacteria, they are most commonly treated with antibiotics or antimicrobials. The type of medication and length of treatment will depend on the patient's symptoms and history. The full course treatment should always be completed for UTIs to make sure that the infection is fully clear and to reduce the risk of antibiotic resistance. UTI symptoms can disappear before the infection has completely gone but that doesn't mean one should stop the medication. Drinking lots of water can also help flush the bacteria from your system. A doctor may prescribe a medication to soothe the pain and a heating pad may also be helpful to reduce abdominal pains.

Studies on the effectiveness of Cranberry juice for preventing or treating UTIs have produced mixed results. The red berry contains tannin that prevents E. coli bacteria from sticking to the walls of the bladder where they can cause infection. However, a 2012 review of 24 studies looking into the effectiveness of cranberry juice or extract on UTIs found they did not significantly reduce the incidence of UTIs.

CHRONIC UTIs

About 1 in 5 women experience a second UTI while some are plagued incessantly. In most cases, the culprit is a different type or strain of bacteria. A group of these renegades invade the body's cells and form a community safe from antibiotics and the immune system. They can travel out of the cells and then re-invade, ultimately establishing a colony of antibiotic-resistant bacteria primed to attack again and again.

Some women are genetically predisposed to UTIs while others have abnormalities in the structure of their Urinary tract that make them more susceptible to infection. Women with diabetes may be at higher risk because their compromised immune systems make them less able to fight infections like UTIs. Other conditions that increase risk include pregnancy, multiple sclerosis, and anything that affects urine flow such as kidney stones, stroke and spinal cord injury.

UTI TREATMENT OPTIONS

If you have 3 or more UTIs a year, ask your doctor to recommend a special treatment plan. Some treatment options include;

Taking a low dose of antibiotics over a longer period to help prevent repeat infections

Taking a single dose of antibiotic after sex which is a common infection trigger

Using an at-home urine kit when symptoms start.

HOW TO PREVENT UTIs

You can prevent getting UTI or another UTI with the following tips;

Empty your bladder frequently as soon as you feel the need to go; don't rush and be sure you have emptied your bladder completely

Wipe from front to back

Drink lots of water

Choose showers over baths

Stay away from feminine hygiene sprays, scented douches and scented bath products-they only increase irritation.

Cleanse your genital area before sex.

Urinate after sex to flush away any bacteria that may have entered your urethra.

If you use a diaphragm, non-lubricated condoms or spermicidal jelly for birth control, consider switching to another method. Diaphragms can increase bacteria growth while non-lubricated condoms and spermicides can cause irritation.

Keep your genital area dry by wearing cotton underwear and loose-fitting clothes. Avoid tight jeans and nylon underwear-they can trap moisture creating the perfect environment for bacteria growth.

CHAPTER FOUR-

UTERINE FIBROID

Uterine fibroids also known as uterine leiomyoma or fibroids are benign smooth muscle tumours of the uterus. Most women have no symptoms while others may have painful or heavy periods. If large enough, they may push on the bladder causing a frequent need to urinate. They are non-cancerous growths of the uterus that often appear during child-bearing years. Uterine fibroids aren't associated with an increased risk of uterine cancer and almost never develop into cancer. Fibroids range in size from seedlings, undetectable by the human eye, to bulky masses that can distort and enlarge the uterus. One can have a single fibroid or multiple ones. In extreme cases, multiple fibroids can expand the uterus so much that it reaches the rib cage.

WHAT CAUSES FIBROID?

While it is not clearly known what causes fibroids, it is believed that each tumour develops from an aberrant muscle cell in the uterus, which multiplies rapidly because of the influence of oestrogen.

WHAT INCREASES ONE'S RISK OF GETTING UTERINE FIBROIDS?

- Age, fibroids become more common as women age, especially from the 30s and 40s through menopause. After menopause, fibroids usually shrink.
- Family history. Having a family member with fibroids increases your risk.
- Obesity

SYMPTOMS OF FIBROIDS

Some women who have fibroids have no symptoms or mild symptoms while other women have more severe, disruptive symptoms. The following are the most common symptoms for uterine fibroids; however, each individual may experience symptoms differently. Some of the uterine fibroids may include;

Heavy or prolonged menstrual periods that can cause anaemia

Abnormal bleeding between menstrual periods

Pelvic pain (caused as tumour presses on pelvic organs)

Frequent urination

Low back pain

Pain during sexual intercourse

A firm mass, often located near the middle of the pelvis, which can be felt by the physician.

HOW ARE FIBROIDS DIAGNOSED?

Fibroids are most often found during a routine pelvic examination. This, along with an abdominal examination, may indicate a firm, irregular pelvic mass to the physician. In addition to a complete medical history and physical and pelvic and/or abdominal examination, diagnostic procedures for uterine fibroids may include:

X-ray

Transvaginal ultrasound also called ultrasonography

Magnetic Resonance Imaging (MRI)

Hysterosalpingography; X-ray examination of the uterus and fallopian tubes that uses dye and is often performed to rule out tubal obstruction

Hysteroscopy; visual examination of the canal of the cervix and the interior of the uterus using a hysteroscope inserted into the vaginal

Endometrial biopsy

TREATMENT OF FIBROIDS

in women whose fibroids are large and causing significant symptoms, treatment may be necessary. Treatment will be determined by your health care provider based on;

Your overall health and medical history

Extent of the disease

Your tolerance for specific medications, procedures or therapies

Expectations for the course of the disease

Your opinion or preference

Your desire for pregnancy

In general, treatment for fibroids may include;

Hysterectomy ; it involves the surgical removal of the entire uterus,

Conservative surgical therapy which uses a procedure called myomectomy. With this approach, physicians will remove the fibroids but leave the uterus intact to enable future pregnancy

Gonadotropin -Releasing Hormone agonists (GnRH agonists); this approach lowers levels of oestrogen and triggers a `medical menopause'. Sometimes, GnRH agonists are used to shrink the fibroid, making surgical treatment easier,

Anti-hormonal agents; certain drugs oppose oestrogen such as progestin and danazol and appear effective in treating fibroids.

Uterine artery embolization also called uterine fibroid embolization is a newer minimally-invasive (without a large abdominal incision) technique. The embolization cuts off the blood supply to the fibroids, thus shrinking them. Health care providers continue to evaluate the long-term implications of this procedure on fertility and regrowth of the fibroid tissue.

Anti-inflammatory painkillers which is often effective for women who experience occasional pelvic pain or discomfort.

CHAPTER FIVE-

PREGNANCY

Pregnancy, also known as gravidity (Latin for heavy) or gestation is the time during which one or more offspring develops inside a woman. They can occur by sexual intercourse or assisted reproductive technology. An embryo is the developing offspring during the first eight weeks following conception, after which, the term, `foetus' is used until birth. Pregnancy is typically divided into three trimesters. The first trimester is from week one through 12 and includes conception. Conception is when the sperm fertilizes the egg. The fertilized egg travels down the fallopian tube and attaches itself to the inside of the uterus, where it begins to form the foetus and placenta. The first trimester carries the highest risk of miscarriage. The second trimester is from week 13 through 28. Around the middle of the second trimester, movement of the foetus may be felt. At 28 weeks, more than 90% of the babies can survive outside of the uterus if provided high-quality medical care. The third trimester is from 29 weeks through 40 weeks.

Pre-natal improves pregnancy outcomes. Pre-natal care may include taking extra folic acid, avoiding drugs and alcohol, regular exercise, blood tests, and regular physical examinations. Complications of pregnancy may include;

High blood pressure of pregnancy

Gestational diabetes

Iron-deficiency anaemia

Severe abdominal pains among others

nausea and vomiting among others

Term pregnancy is 37 to 41 weeks with early term being 37 and 38 weeks, full term being 39 and 40 weeks and late term being 41 weeks. After 41 weeks, it is known as post term. Babies born before 37 weeks are preterm and are at higher risk of health problems such as cerebral palsy. Delivery before 39 weeks by labour induction or caesarean section is not recommended unless required for other medical reasons.

Nutrition during pregnancy is important to ensure healthy growth of the foetus and pregnant women are counseled on the particular foods to eat and avoid. Most women can continue to engage in sexual activities throughout pregnancy. Most research suggests that during pregnancy, both sexual desire and frequency of sexual relations decrease. Sex during pregnancy is low-risk behaviour except when the healthcare provider advises that sexual intercourse be avoided for particular medical reasons. Regular aerobic exercise during pregnancy does not only maintain physical fitness but does appear to decrease the risk of Caesarean section.

SIGNS AND SYMPTOMS OF PREGNANCY

The symptoms or discomforts of pregnancy are those conditions that arise as a result of the pregnancy but pose no threat to the activities of daily living or the health of the mother or child. This is in contrast to pregnancy complications. Some discomforts can be considered complications when they become very severe. For example, nausea can be a discomfort, but if, in combination with significant vomiting, causes water-electrolyte imbalance, it is a complication. Common signs, symptoms and discomforts of pregnancy are;

- Tiredness
- Constipation
- Pelvic girdle pain
- Back pain
- Swelling
- Increased urinary frequency
- Urinary Tract Infection
- Varicose veins
- Haemorrhoids (piles)
- Regurgitation, heartburn and nausea
- Pregnancy-related stretch marks
- Breast tenderness
- Missed menstrual period
- Linea nigra (pigmentation of the linea alba) thus darkening of the skin in a midline of the abdomen
- Increased basal body temperature sustained for over 2 weeks after ovulation
- Darkening of the cervix, vagina and vulva (Chadwick's sign)
- Softening of the vaginal portion of the cervix (Goodell's sign)
- Darkening of the nipples and areolas due to an increase in hormones

Aside the signs, pregnancy can be detected by having a pregnancy test.

SUDDEN INFANT DEATH SYNDROME (SIDS)

SIDS is the unexplained death, usually during sleep, of a seemingly healthy baby less than a year old. SIDS is sometimes known as crib death because the infants often die in their cribs. Although the cause is unknown, it appears that SIDS may be associated with abnormalities in the portion of an infant's brain that controls breathing and arousal from sleep. Researchers have discovered some factors that may put babies at extra risk and have identified some measures that could protect the child and one of the most important measure if not the most important measure is to place babies on their back to sleep. Other measures are;

To prevent smothering or suffocation, always lay your baby down to sleep on either a firm mattress or surface in a crib.. the bed should be firm with fitted sheets without blankets, pillows, sheepskin, stuffed toys or crib bumpers.

Don't smoke around your baby

Keep your sleeping baby close but not in your bed-keep them in their cribs

Breastfeed your baby as long as you can

Immunize your baby

Keep your baby from overheating; dress them in light, comfortable clothes for sleeping and keep the room temperature at a level that's comfortable for an adult.

Don't give honey to an infant under 1 year old

BIRTH DEFECTS

While in the womb, some babies have problems with how their organs and body parts form, how they work or how their bodies turn food into energy. These health problems are called birth defects. There are more than 4,000 different kinds of birth defects, ranging from minor ones that need no treatment to serious ones that cause disabilities or require medical or surgical treatment. If a baby is born with a part of the body that is missing or malformed, it is called a structural birth defect. Heart defects are the most common type of structural defect. Others include spina bifida, cleft palate, clubfoot, and congenital dislocated hip. When there is a problem with a baby's body chemistry, it is called a metabolic birth defect. Metabolic defects prevent the body from properly breaking down food to create energy. Examples of metabolic defects include Tay-sachs disease, a fatal disease that affects the central nervous system, and Phenylketonuria (PKU), which affects the way the body processes protein.

 For people who want to become parents, it's important to know that some birth defects can be prevented. During a woman's pregnancy, taking folic acid and getting enough iodine in the diet can help prevent some types of birth defects but it is also important to realize that most babies born with birth defects are born to two healthy parents with no obvious health problems or risk factors.

CAUSES OF BIRTH DEFECTS

Environmental causes; if a mother has certain infections such as Toxoplasmosis during pregnancy, her baby can have a birth defect. Other conditions that cause defects include Rubella and Chickenpox. Also, alcohol abuse by the mother may cause Fetal Alcohol Syndrome and certain medicines taken by the mother can also cause birth defects.

Genital causes; every cell in the body has chromosomes containing genes that determine a person's unique characteristics. During conception, a child inherits one of each pair of chromosomes (and one of each pair of the genes they contain) from each parent. An error during the process can cause a baby to be born with too few or too many chromosomes or with a damaged chromosome. One well-known birth defect caused by a chromosome problem is Down syndrome. A baby develops Down syndrome after getting one extra chromosome. Other genetic defects happen when both parents pass along a faulty gene for the same disease; this is called recessive inheritance and includes conditions such as Tay-Sachs disease and cystic fibrosis.

A disease or defect can also happen when only one parent passes on the gene for that disease. This is called dominant inheritance and includes birth defects such as Achondroplasia (a form of dwarfism) and Marfan syndrome (a disorder characterized by abnormally long fingers, arms and legs). Also, some boys inherit disorders from genes passed on to them only by their mothers. These defects which include conditions like Haemophilia, and colour blindness are called X-linked because the genes are carried on the X chromosome.

COMMON BIRTH DEFECTS

Some common birth defects are;

Cleft lip and/or palate; it happens when the tissues of the mouth or lip don't form properly during foetal development, leaving an opening, division, or split in that area. A cleft lip is a long opening between the upper lip and the nose whereas a cleft palate is an opening between the roof of the mouth and the nasal cavity. Clefting can be surgically repaired.

Cerebral palsy; it is considered a neurological disorder caused by a non-progressive brain injury or malformation that occurs while the child's brain is under development. It primarily affects body movement and muscle coordination. It has no cure but can be managed.

Foetal Alcohol Syndrome (FAS); it causes slowed growth, intellectual disability, abnormalities in facial features and problems with the central nervous system. It cannot be cured or treated but can be prevented by avoiding alcohol intake during pregnancy.

Neutral Tube Defects (NTD); this normally happens in the first month of the pregnancy when the structure that develops into the brain and spinal cord is forming. Normally, this structure folds into a tube by the 29th day after conception. When the tube doesn't close completely, the baby has an NTD. The two most common forms of this defects are Spina bifida which happens when the spinal column doesn't close completely around the spinal cord and Anencephaly which involves the lack of development of parts of the brain.

Heart defects which include; Atrial and Ventricular Septal defects (holes in the walls that separate the heart into its left and right sides), Patent Ductus Arteriosus (happens when the tubular blood channel that allows the blood to bypass the lungs while the baby is in the womb doesn't close as expected after birth), Coarctation of the Aorta (narrowing of the aorta), transposition of the great Arteries, hypoplastic left heart system and tetralogy of Fallot (combination of four heart defects that involves restriction in the flow of blood to the lungs). Although the specific cause of most heart defects isn't known, it is known to health practitioners that many defects happen during the first trimester of the pregnancy. Exposure to certain medications such as chemotherapy drugs, thalidomide and anti-seizure drug phenytoin during the first trimester of the pregnancy may play a role in causing heart defects. Other causes include maternal alcohol abuse, rubella or German measles infection and diabetes during pregnancy.

Gastrointestinal Tract defects; structural defects that can happen at any point along the gastrointestinal tract which is made up of the oesophagus, stomach, small and large intestines, rectum and anus. The incomplete or abnormal development of any of these organs can cause blockages that can lead to swallowing difficulties, vomiting, and problems with bowel movements. Some of these defects are oesophageal atresia, diaphragmatic hernia, pyloric stenosis, Hirsch sprung disease, anal atresia, biliary atresia, gastroschisis and omphalocele among others.

Genetic birth defects; such as Cystic Fibrosis (CF) which affects cells in the lining of the skin and many passageways in the lungs, digestive system and reproductive system sand causes these body parts to produce a thick, sticky mucus, Down syndrome, Fragile X syndrome which causes mental impairment that ranges from learning disabilities to intellectual disabilities, autistic behaviours and problems with attention and hyperactivity, Muscular Dystrophy which is a general term used to describe more than 40 different types of muscle diseases, Phenylketonuria

(PKU) which affects the way the body processes protein and can cause intellectual disability, sickle cell disease, Tay-Sachs disease and etc.

INFECTIONS THAT CAUSE BIRTH DEFECTS

Infections during pregnancy can cause a variety of birth defects. Some of these infections include;

Congenital Rubella syndrome; it poses the highest risk of foetal damage. A child can have vision and/or hearing loss, heart defects, intellectual disability and cerebral palsy as a result of this infection.

Cytomegalovirus (CMV); it's probably the most common infection that shows up at birth. If a pregnant woman gets this infection, her child may have low birth weight, mental retardation or learning disabilities and hearing loss.

Toxoplasmosis; this infection can cause eye infections that threaten vision, hearing loss, learning disabilities, enlarged liver or spleen, mental retardation and cerebral palsy in babies born by infected pregnant women.

Genital herpes virus; infection of the mother can cause brain damage, cerebral palsy, vision or hearing impairment and death of the baby if the virus is transmitted to the infant before or during the birth. Herpes complications are most commonly due to infection during the birth process and are not commonly classified as birth defects.

Congenital varicella syndrome; it is caused by chicken pox and can lead to scars, defects of muscle and bone, malformed and paralyzed limbs, a smaller-than-normal head, blindness, seizures, and intellectual disability. This is a rare occurrence in pregnant women who become infected with chicken pox.

Congenital syphilis; in early congenital syphilis, a child may be born prematurely or have an enlarged liver or spleen, inflammation of the nasal cartilage or bone changes and central nervous system problems. A child with late congenital syphilis may have abnormalities of the facial bones and teeth, vision problems and deafness.

Women who are pregnant should talk to their health care providers about ways to avoid these infections and what to do if they are exposed to them. Pregnant women must attend pre-natal and post-natal sessions since many birth defects are diagnosed even before a baby is born through prenatal tests. Prenatal tests can also help determine if a mother has an infection or other conditions that is dangerous for the foetus. Others birth defects that can't be detected before birth can be identified during routine new-born screenings.

PREVENTING BIRTH DEFECTS

Many birth defects can't be prevented but a woman can do some things before and during pregnancy to help lower the chances of having a baby with a birth defect. Before pregnancy, women should;

Make sure their vaccinations are up to date

Make sure they don't have any Sexually Transmitted Diseases/Infections (STDs/STIs)

Get the daily recommended dose of folic acid before trying to conceive

Avoid unnecessary medicines and talk to their doctor about medicines they are taking.

If there's a family history of birth defects or the pregnant woman is part of a high-risk group (due to age, ethnic background, or medical history), she should consider meeting with a genetic counsellor to determine her baby's risk. During pregnancy, it's important to take prenatal vitamins and eat a healthy diet in addition to take the following precaution;

Don't smoke and avoid second-hand smoke

Don't drink alcohol

Avoid all illicit drugs

Exercise and get plenty of rest

Get early and regular prenatal care

By following these pregnancy precautions, women can help reduce their babies' risk of birth defects.

CHAPTER SIX-

SEXUALLY TRANSMITTED INFECTIONS/DISEASES (STIs/STDs)

Sexually Transmitted Infections (STIs), also known as Sexually Transmitted Diseases (STDs) or Venereal Diseases (VD), are diseases that are passed on from one person to the other through sexual contact, and sometimes by genital contact-The infection can be passed on via vaginal intercourse, oral sex and anal sex. Some STIs can spread through the use of unsterilized IV drug needles, from mother to baby during childbirth or breastfeeding and blood transfusions. Microorganisms that exist on the skin or mucus membranes of the male or female genital area can be transmitted, as can organisms in semen, vaginal secretions or blood during sexual intercourse.

The term, `Venereal Disease' is much less used today while STDs is slowly giving way to STIs because STIs has a broader range of meaning thus a person can pass on the infection without having a disease-meaning they do not have to be ill to infect other people. Examples of STIs include;

- Chlamydia
- Chancroid
- Crabs (pubic lice)
- Genital herpes
- Genital warts
- Hepatitis B
- HIV/AIDS
- Human Papillomavirus (HPV)
- Trichomoniasis (parasitic infection)
- Molluscum Contagiosum
- Pelvic Inflammatory Disease (PID)
- Scabies
- Syphilis
- Gonorrhoea
- Yeast infections

The World Health Organisation (WHO) estimated over ten years ago that over 1 million people each day become infected with a STI- most experts believe that the figure is considerably high today, majority of these infections occur in young adults aged up to 25 years while approximately one-third occur among individuals younger than 20 years of age. Globally, girls aged 14 to 19 are almost twice more susceptible than boys of the same age.

STIs IN WOMEN

Many STIs don't show symptoms at all in women but some common symptoms of an STI can include:

- Vaginal itching
- Rashes or sores
- Unusual vaginal discharge
- Pain during sex
- Changes in urination which includes frequent urination and burning sensation during urination
- Abnormal bleeding

STIs can lead to fertility problems and an increased risk of cervical cancer if left untreated. These risks make it more important to practice safe sex. Every year worldwide, there are approximately 357 million new infections of syphilis, chlamydia, gonorrhoea and trichomoniasis. Due to the fact that many women don't show symptoms with some STIs, they may not know they need treatment. Some of the most common STIs in women include:

- Human Papillomavirus (HPV)
- Gonorrhoea
- Chlamydia
- Genital herpes

HPV is the most common STI in women and it is also the main cause of cervical cancer. A vaccine is available that can help prevent against strains of HPV. Gonorrhoea and chlamydia are common bacteria STIs. Genital herpes is also a common STI.

PREVENTION

Get tested regularly

Use protection during sex

Honest communication with your sexual partner and doctor about your sexual history is really important.

Don't keep multiple sex partners since it keeps you at risk

Get vaccinated. Vaccines are available to prevent HPV, Hepatitis A and Hepatitis B.

WHAT TO DO AFTER YOU HAVE BEEN DIAGNOSED

Start any treatment your doctor prescribes for you immediately

Contact your partner(s) and let them know that they need to get tested and treated too

Abstain from sex until your infection is either cured or until your doctor gives approval

CHAPTER SEVEN

TURNER SYNDROME

Turner syndrome is a chromosomal condition that affects development in females. The most common feature of Turner syndrome is short stature, which becomes evident by age 5. An early loss of ovarian function is also very common. The ovaries develop normally at first but egg cells usually die prematurely and most ovarian tissue degenerates before birth. Many affected girls do no undergo puberty unless they receive hormone therapy and most are unable to conceive. A small percentage of girls with Turner syndrome retain normal ovarian function through young adulthood. About 30% of females with Turner syndrome have extra folds of skin on the neck (webbed neck), a low hairline at the back of the neck, puffiness or swelling (lymphedema) of the hands and feet, skeletal abnormalities or kidney problems and one-third to one-half of individuals with Turner syndrome are born with a heart defect, such as a narrowing of the large artery leaving the heart (coarctation of the aorta) or abnormalities of the valve that connects the aorta with the heart (the aortic valve). Complications associated with these heart defects can be life-threatening. Most girls and women with Turner syndrome have normal intelligence. Developmental delays, non-verbal learning disabilities and behavioural problems are possible, although these characteristics vary among affected individuals.

Turner syndrome was first discovered in 1938 by Dr. Henry Turner but chromosomal abnormalities were not discovered until 1960. Dr. Turner was an Endocrinologist, from Oklahoma City, who discovered this syndrome when a group of women he was treating for dwarfism didn't respond to treatments.

HOW DOES IT HAPPEN?

Most girls are born with two X chromosomes but girls with Turner syndrome are born with only one X chromosome. The effects vary widely among girls with Turner syndrome. It all depends on how many of the body's cells are affected by the changes to the X chromosome.

OTHER EFFECTS OF TURNER SYNDROME

A number of other health problems occur more often in girls with Turner syndrome including:

- Kidney problems
- High blood pressure
- Heart problems
- Overweight
- Hearing difficulties
- Diabetes
- Thyroid problems
- Learning difficulties particularly in math
- May have a hard time with tasks that require skills such as map reading or visual organization
- Differently shaped ears that are set lower on the sides of the head than usual
- Abnormal bone development especially the bones of the hands and elbows
- A larger than usual number of moles on the skin
- Edema (extra fluid) in the hands and feet
- Because Turner syndrome can affect how a girl looks, it normally results in developing a low self-esteem.

TREATING TURNER SYNDROME

Turner syndrome is a condition that is caused by a chromosomal abnormality and therefore, there is no cure. However, scientists have developed a number of treatments which include;

Help with growth problems with growth hormone

Oestrogen replacement which helps develop physical changes during puberty including breast development and menstrual periods

In Vitro fertilization can make it possible for some women with Turner syndrome to become pregnant

CHAPTER EIGHT

RETT SYNDROME

Rett syndrome (RTT), originally termed cerebroatropic hyperammonemia is a rare genetic postnatal neurological disorder of the grey matter of the brain that almost exclusively affects females but has also been found in male patients. It is usually discovered in the first two years of life. The clinical features include small hands and feet and a deceleration of the rate of head growth including microcephaly in some. Repetitive stereotyped hand movements such as wringing and/or repeatedly putting hands into the mouth are also noted. People with RTT are prone to gastrointestinal disorders and up to 80% have seizures. They typically have no verbal skills and about 50% of affected individuals do not walk. Scoliosis, growth failure and constipation are very common and can be problematic. The signs of this disorder are mostly easily confused with those of Angelman syndrome, cerebral palsy and autism. Rett syndrome occurs in approximately 1:10,000 live female births in all geographies and across all ethnicities.

The syndrome was first discovered by an Austrian neurologist, Andreas Rett in 1966. While the disorder was identified scientifically and could be reliably diagnosed, the causes remained unknown for decades. Huda Zoghbi demonstrated in 1999 that mutations in the gene, MECP2, cause Rett syndrome. Prior to the discovery of a genetic cause, Rett syndrome had been arbitrarily designated as a pervasive developmental disorder by the Diagnostic and Statistical Manual of Mental Disorders which is published by the American Psychiatric Association (APA) together with the autism spectrum disorders. Some argued against this conclusive assignment because RTT resembles non-autistic disorders such as Fragile X syndrome, Down syndrome or Tuberous Sclerosis that exhibit autistic features coincidentally. After research proved the molecular mechanism, in 2013 the DSM-5 (Diagnostic and Statistical Manual of Mental Disorders, Fifth Edition) removed the syndrome altogether from classification as a mental disorder.

SIGNS AND SYMPTOMS

The age when symptoms appear varies but most babies with Rett syndrome seem to grow normally for the first 6 months before any signs of the disorder are obvious. The most common changes usually show up when babies are between 12 and 18 months and they can be sudden or progress slowly. Some signs and symptoms include:

- Slowed growth
- Problems with hand movements
- No language skills
- Problems with muscles and coordination
- Trouble with breathing; a child with Rett syndrome may have uncoordinated breathing and seizures including very fast breathing.

There are some signs of Rett syndrome that are similar to autism which include:

- Incontinence
- Screaming fits
- Inconsolable crying
- Breath holding, hyperventilation and air swallowing
- Avoidance of eye contact
- Markedly impaired use of non-verbal behaviours to regulate social interaction
- Loss of speech
- Sensory problems
- Sleep regression
- Signs of RTT that are also present in cerebral palsy include;
- Possible short stature
- Hypotonia
- Delayed or absent ability to walk
- Gait/movement difficulties
- Ataxia
- Microcephaly in some
- Gastrointestinal problems
- Some forms of spasticity
- Dystonia
- Chorea which is the spasmodic movements of hand or facial muscles
- Bruxism or grinding of teeth

CAUSES

Most children with Rett syndrome have a mutation in the gene MECP2 located on the X chromosome and can arise sporadically or form germline mutations. In less than 10% of RTT cases, mutations in the genes CDKL5 or FOXG1 have also been found to resemble it. Although Rett syndrome is genetic, children almost never inherit the faulty gene from their parents. Rather, it's a chance mutation that happens in the DNA. When boys develop this disorder, they rarely live past birth because males have only one X chromosome instead of two in girls so the effects of the disease are much more serious and almost fatal.

TREATMENTS

Although there is no cure for Rett syndrome, there are treatments that can improve symptoms and children should continue these treatments for their entire life. The best options available to treat Rett syndrome include:

- Standard medical care and medication
- Physical therapy
- Speech therapy
- Occupational therapy
- Good nutrition
- Behavioural therapy
- Supportive services

CHAPTER NINE

CERVICAL CANCER

Cervical cancer is a cancer that begins in the uterine cervix, the lower end of the uterus that contracts the upper vagina. It is due to the abnormal growth of cells that have the ability to invade or spread to other parts of the body. It can often be treated when found early. It is usually found at a very early stage through a Pap test. Early on, typically no symptoms are seen. Later, symptoms may include abnormal vaginal bleeding, pelvic pain or pain during sexual intercourse. Human Papillomavirus (HPV) infection appears to be involved in the development of more than 90% of cases thus most cervical cancer is caused by HPV though not all types of HPV can cause cervical cancer. Other risk factors include smoking, a weak immune system, birth control pills, starting sex at a young age and having many sexual partners but these are less important. Diagnosis is typically by cervical screening followed by a biopsy. Medical imaging is then done to determine whether or not cancer has spread.

HPV vaccines protect against between two and seven high risk of this family of viruses and may prevent up to 90% of cervical cancers. As a risk of cancer still exists, guidelines recommend continuing regular Pap smears. Worldwide, cervical cancer is both the fourth most common cause of cancer and the fourth most common cause of death from cancer in women. In 2012, an estimated 528,000 cases of cervical cancer occurred with 266,000 deaths. About 70% of cervical cancers occur in developing countries.

Two vaccines, Gardasil and Cervarix are vaccines that are available to prevent HPV infection.

SIGNS AND SYMPTOMS

The early stages of cervical cancer may be completely free of symptoms. Vaginal bleeding, contact bleeding (one most common form being bleeding after sexual intercourse) or rarely a vaginal mass may indicate the presence of malignancy. Also, moderate pain during sexual intercourse and vaginal discharge are symptoms of cervical cancer. Symptoms of advanced cervical cancer may include:

- Loss of appetite
- Weight loss
- Fatigue
- Pelvic pain
- Back pain
- Leg pain

- Swollen legs
- Heavy vaginal bleeding
- Bone fractures
- Rarely leakage of urine or faeces from the vagina
- Bleeding after douching or after a pelvic exam is a common symptom of cervical cancer
- Bleeding after going through menopause
- Bleeding or spotting between periods
- Longer or heavier menstrual periods than usual

TREATMENT

The treatment of cervical cancer varies worldwide largely due to access to surgeons skilled in radical pelvic surgery and the emergence of "fertility-sparing therapy" in developed nations. Because cervical cancers are radio-sensitive, radiation may be used in all stages where surgical options still exist. Surgical intervention may have better outcomes than radiological approaches. Treatment options for cervical cancer include:

- Radiation therapy
- Surgery
- Chemotherapy
- Targeted therapy

CHAPTER TEN

BREAST CANCER

Breast cancer is cancer that develops from the breast tissue. About 5-10% of cases are due to genes inherited from a person's parents including BRCA1 and BRCA2 among others. Breast cancer most commonly develops in cells from the lining of milk ducts and the lobules that supply the ducts with milk. Cancers developing from the ducts are known as ductal carcinomas, while those developing from lobules are known as lobular carcinomas. In addition, there are more than 18 other sub-types of breast cancer. Some cancers such as ductal carcinoma in situ develop from pre-invasive lesions. The diagnosis of breast cancer is confirmed by taking a biopsy of the concerning lump. Once the diagnosis is made, further tests are done to determine if the cancer has spread beyond the breast and which treatments it may respond to. Outcomes for breast cancer vary depending on the cancer type, extent of disease and person's age. Survival rates in the world are poorer in developing countries as compared to the developed. Worldwide, breast cancer is the leading type of cancer in women, accounting for 25% of all cases. In 2012, it resulted in 1.68 million cases and 522,000 deaths. Research shows that it is more common in developed countries and is more than 100 times more common in women than in men.

SIGNS AND SYMPTOMS

- Lump in breast
- Lumps or swelling in the armpit or pain in the armpits
- Pitting or redness of the skin of the breast
- A rash around or on one of the nipples
- An area of thickened tissue in breast
- Changes in the appearance of the nipple; it may become sunken or inverted
- The size or shape of the breast changes
- Peeling, scaling or flaking of the nipple-skin or breast skin
- Discharge from the nipples
- Constant pain in part of the breast

RISK FACTORS

Risk factors can be divided into two categories such as:

Modifiable risk factors; factors that people can change by themselves such as consumption of alcoholic beverages, smoking tobacco, dietary factors such as a high fat diet and obesity-related high cholesterol levels. Dietary iodine, low fibre intake, radiation and shift-work.

Fixed risk factors: things that cannot be changed such as age, biological sex. The primary risk factors for breast cancer are being female and older age. Other potential risk factors include genetics, lack of childbearing or lack of breastfeeding, higher levels of certain hormones and etc. Recent studies have indicated that exposure to light pollution is a risk factor for the development of breast cancer.

PREVENTION

The following steps can be taken to reduce risks of getting breast cancer:

- Limit alcohol intake
- No smoking
- Weight control
- Be physically active
- Breast-feed
- Avoid exposure to radiation and environmental pollution

TREATMENT

- Surgery
- Radiation therapy
- Chemotherapy
- Systemic therapy
- Hormonal therapy
- Targeted therapy

CHAPTER ELEVEN-

DEPRESSION

Depression is a state of low mood and aversion to activity that can affect a person's thoughts, behaviour, feelings and sense of well-being. Depressed mood is a feature of some psychiatric syndromes such as major depressive order and dysthymia but it may also be a normal temporal reaction to life events such as bereavement, broken heart, and a symptom of some bodily ailments or a side effect of some drugs and medical treatments, general loss, disappointment, frustrations, among others.

People with a depressed mood can feel sad, anxious, empty, hopeless, helpless, worthless, guilty, irritable, angry, ashamed or restless. They may lose interest in activities that were once pleasurable, experience loss of appetite, or overeating (I normally stuff my mouth with chocolate and biscuits when I'm depressed and trying to stop myself from crying), having problems concentrating, remembering details or making decisions, experience relationship difficulties and may contemplate, attempt or commit suicide. Insomnia, excessive sleeping, fatigue, aches, pains, digestive problems or reduced energy may also be present.

Depression knows not wealth, gender, status or social standing- anyone can be depressed at any point in time of our life but it is up to us to shake it off and move on without it killing us. Depression is different from normal sadness in that, it engulfs your day-to-day life, interfering with your ability to work, study, eat, sleep, have fun and carry out tasks or activities you could have carried out on a normal day. So many issues can end us up in depression include frustration, disappointment, broken heart, inability to hit a set target, blackmail, threats among others and as I said earlier, if we allow depression to engulf us, it ruins our life- it is up to us to always look at the brighter side of things and shake it off.

SYMPTOMS OF DEPRESSION

Depression varies from one person to another but there are some common signs and symptoms. It is important to remember that, these symptoms can be part of life's normal lows but the more symptoms you have, the stronger they are and the longer they have lasted, the more likely it is that you are dealing with depression. Depression often varies according to age and gender with symptoms differing between men and women, or young people and older adults.

Depressed men are less likely to acknowledge feelings of self-loathing and hopelessness. Instead, they tend to complain about fatigue, irritability, sleep problems and loss of interest in work and hobbies. They are also more likely to experience symptoms such as anger, frustration, reckless behaviour and substance abuse whereas women are more likely to experience symptoms such as pronounced feelings of guilt, excessive sleeping, overeating and loss of appetite resulting on either weight loss or gain and constant crying. Depression in women is also impacted by hormonal factors during menstruation, pregnancy, and menopause. Up to 1 in 7 women experience depression following childbirth, a condition known as Postpartum depression. Irritability, anger and agitation are mostly the most noticeable symptoms in depressed teens whereas older adults tend to complain more about the physical rather than the emotional signs like fatigue, unexplained aches and pains and memory problems. Some of the symptoms of depression include:

- Feelings of helplessness and hopelessness
- Loss of interest in daily activities
- Appetite loss or gain leading to significant weight loss or gain
- Sleep changes
- Anger or irritability
- Loss of energy
- Self-loathing; strong feelings of worthlessness or guilt. You harshly criticize yourself for perceived faults and mistakes
- Reckless behaviour such as substance abuse, compulsive gambling, reckless driving or dangerous sport
- Concentration problems
- Unexplained aches and pains

DEPRESSION AND SUICIDE RISK

Depression is a major risk factor for suicide. The deep despair and hopelessness that goes along with depression can make suicide feel like the only way to escape the pain. I remember when I attempted suicide thrice in my teenage days because of mistreatment from certain people, feeling of dejection due to the growing distance between my mum and I, constant judgment from people around me and me constantly blamed for everything making me feel like I am no good amongst others. I remember when I had a car accident on an errand for a neighbour- I was crossing the road when I was knocked by a car. I was only 10 and I knew I was only being respectful by running errands for the elderly and definitely no one sees the future but I was constantly blamed for this accident which got me depressed but as I said earlier, it is up to us to allow ourselves to be swallowed by our problems- just shake them off.

If you have a loved one with depression, take any suicidal talk or behaviour seriously and watch for the warning signs:

- Talking about killing or harming one's self
- Expressing strong feelings of hopelessness or being trapped
- An unusual preoccupation with death or dying
- Acting recklessly as if they have a death wish
- Calling or visiting people to say goodbye
- Getting affairs in order like sudden preparation of will, giving away prized possessions, tying up loose ends and etc
- Saying things like, "everyone will be better off without me" or "I want out" or "I am tired and want to end it all"
- A sudden switch from being extremely depressed to acting calm and happy

If you know of anyone considering suicide, express your opinion and seek help immediately. Don't judge them but try to let them know you understand their state and talk them out of it by making them see the brighter side of things while letting them know how you love and cherish them. It is very good to constantly use the "I love you" words for others to know how important they are to you. Trust me, aside the unusual fashion of some men just using these words without meaning them just to get into the pants of women, these words heal a lot. Talking openly about suicidal thoughts and feelings can save a life.

DEPRESSION CAUSES AND RISK FACTORS

- Loneliness and isolation
- Lack of social support
- Recent stressful life experiences
- Family history of depression
- Marital or relationship problems
- Financial strain
- Early childhood trauma or abuse
- Alcohol or drug abuse
- Unemployment or underemployment
- Health problems or chronic pain

WHAT TO DO WHEN DEPRESSED

- Reach out to people
- Get moving
- Eat a mood boosting diet such as omega-3 fatty acids or even, your favourite meal
- Find ways to engage again with the world
- Seek professional help if support from family and friends and positive lifestyle changes are not enough

PART FOUR-

YOU ARE ON YOUR OWN

CHAPTER ONE-

DEVELOP YOURSELF

Personal development covers activities that improve awareness and identity, develop talents and potential, build human capital and facilitate employability, enhance the quality of life and contribute to the realization of dreams and aspirations. Many people are caught up in the race of this world- they seem so busy that they forget themselves and forget to spend time with themselves. It is extremely important to find time for yourselves and spend time with yourself because it offers individuals an opportunity to gain some perspective about their lives so that they may begin planning for their futures. Self-development is a process whereby individuals evaluate their own lives, observe the personal growth they have experienced and decide whether they are satisfied or not.

Everyone is troubled or plagued by one problem or the other. Regardless of whether you are a male or female, rich or poor, good-looking or not, happy or not, we are likely to encounter problems that could pertain either to our future or our past. Such problems can either turn into stumbling blocks or obstacles or motivation if manages effectively. However, the problem is that many people are not aware of the fact that they can exert control over their own minds, and maximize their potential.

WHAT SELF-DEVELOPMENT DEALS WITH

Reconciling conflict/ Reconciling with your past; one can never move on in life if they still carry a heavy backpack of their past with them. You don't have to let go of your past in order to move on but instead, you have to reconcile with your past. These two, "letting go" and "reconciling" are two different things altogether. You can let go of something by simply dropping it but that doesn't end it because it may later come back staring at you but when you reconcile with your past, you understand situations or experiences better, you face every emotion, thrash things out and make peace- meaning that the issue is done and dusted and is no longer a heavy cross.

The process of self-development is deeply concerned with resolving emotional conflicts and issues that you may have with yourself and others. Self-loathing comes as a result of a lot of hanging issues we have with ourselves and others and until these issues are reconciled, we do not have a complete peace of mind to move on which becomes a big hindrance or obstacle to us developing ourselves. Learn to forgive yourself and others, keeping in mind that there is none perfect and to err is human. It is very easy to fall prey to our own emotions and past unresolved conflicts and these sometimes kill our confidence and make us insecure and confused about the next step to take in life. To be able to develop ourselves, we need to reconcile with our past and conflicts- wear off that heavy backpack.

Finding Meaning; you can't do things you don't understand neither can you believe in things you have no idea about. Until you find meaning to every situation or experience, you cannot understand why things happen and what meaning those experiences bring to your life. Give your life a meaning- find meaning to your existence as a person and to your experiences and this can help you in developing yourself. Until you know yourself, your capabilities, your fears and etc, you can never take a step higher.

Be understanding and compassionate; until you understand yourself and pamper yourself with a little compassion in that, you support your inner being and be empathetic to yourself for decisions you make, and you will keep being hard on yourself for nothing. Also, when you learn to understand others and be empathetic to them, you can't also have inner peace or a good relationship with others because you will constantly worry about or fight about issues you could have easily brushed off. One thing you should know is that man is never an island and therefore can easily be corrupted or influenced by the actions of others. Keep a free-mind and try to understand everyone for what they do including what you do yourself.

Grow Confidence; you can't survive in a world of billions of people if you don't have confidence. You can't move on in life if you are not confident. You must be able to face yourself before you can face the world. Showing confidence is never about being confident to the world- you can't show confidence to the world when you in the first place cannot be confident to yourself. To be able to develop yourself, you must be confident in yourself, push the limits of your potential and challenge yourself. Never allow your mistakes to affect you.

FIND YOURSELF

You cannot develop yourself until you find yourself- until you find yourself, you will continue to be confused about what really you want to be or you want in life. Let me tell you a story about myself. I am a one in a million child who instead of developing a low self-esteem and low confidence level in certain situations; the situations rather raise my libido against these two. I am inspired by hatred and opposition. I get challenged and propelled to rise and get things done when I am run down by people or thought of to be unqualified or said to be of no good. I actually gather momentum from these and that means, I know myself and I know what triggers me to work harder. You have to find yourself- know what breaks or strengthens you, know what you want in life before you can develop yourself.

I still remember my usual response to my dad's question about what I wanted to be when I grow. I was just 8 then but my usual response was, "I want to be a magistrate and a journalist"- I didn't know how I was going to combine the two though but I always said that. I got to senior high school and I lost myself in the early years or probably I just wanted to explore many options and opportunities. I was brought up in strict homes where you barely had friends or went out so probably, it was the joy from the liberty I had in school that brought about few changes. I started rapping and developed this sudden tom boy attitude but in my mind, I still wanted to be that magistrate but here I was losing myself because there was no one to guide me. I switched schools and in my new environment, I found myself and dropped all these and became focused again. I later came to the university and I almost got carried away because I found the freedom I never had at home in abundance in the university. Here I was where no one could seize my phone even though I started using a phone after senior high, or lock me up in the house- I was at liberty to do whatever I wanted and this made me want to try all the experiences I missed. I had never gone out to parties or a club or had this freedom before and I wanted to experience them all. I went to the club about three times just to experience what goes on there and got a bit distracted about what I really wanted- started rapping again and I almost lost myself because I couldn't handle what I had just seen.

I later in level 200, realized and said to myself, `this is not what I want to be, I don't want to end up in any entertainment industry. I still want to be that magistrate'. I realized I had veered off my course for a while and fortunately for me, I spoke to myself and found myself and I am happy I did.

Most times, we end up in careers or occupations or marriages or overall situations because we lost ourselves along the line. Not all of us will be lucky to have people as guides as I didn't have any myself because I discovered by myself that I had veered off and went back on track, but I believe we know ourselves better and we only know what we really and truly want. We have to discover ourselves and find out who we are and where we want to be lest we keep getting lost. To be able to achieve your dream and be what you want to be, you must find yourself.

NOTHING MUST BE A HINDRANCE TO YOU DEVELOPING YOURSELF

Nothing must be a hindrance to you developing yourself and when I say nothing, I mean nothing not even yourself. Most often, we allow certain things to hinder us from reaching our dreams but I believe that if we truly have dreams, we must achieve them and nothing should be a hindrance. There may be hurdles but we must be prepared to jump above those hurdles to reach to our dreams. A dream will continue to be just a dream until we wake up, realize it and make it a living legacy. Breath unto that dream, put life in it but you can only do that by working hard to achieve it.

Your gender must never be a hindrance to your success. Never! This is because, one's gender doesn't incapacitate them. We only incapacitate ourselves by belittling our abilities and not believing in ourselves and our worth. Haven't you seen other women out there doing it and succeeding? So why should you be moved by an immature statement that you are a woman and so, you can't do it. Is a woman not equally human like a man? Doesn't she have same five senses? So what are you talking about? Get out there and succeed.

Your geographical location should never be a hindrance to your success. Shine in whichever corner that you are- you don't need a bigger platform to show how big you are or your worth because your worth is in your mind. You are what you think of yourself and not what others think of you. You can only succeed if you believe in your potentials and abilities. If you always consider what others will say, you will end up losing yourself and your dreams. When I was taken to Antoa senior high school from St. John's Grammar, initially I felt sad and broken and it got to a time that I even wanted to stop schooling but I got motivated in the fact that, it didn't really matter where I was, my life depended on my life choices and what I was ready to make out of experiences and every situation. And when I did, I shone in that little corner. I led the school to competitions and made unprecedented successful stories. It only took me to realize that, where I was didn't really matter to be successful. Never be discouraged by whatever situation or environment you find yourself in but instead, be inspired by difficult moments to strive harder so that in future, your story can be a motivation or an inspirational guide to others.

CHAPTER TWO-

MARRIAGE IS NEVER A CAREER

I get really sad when I hear statements like, "I am a woman and I don't need much hard work, all I need is a rich husband", "after my first degree, what next?-to marry of course", "a woman's value is determined by the man she marries". Omg! This is serious! How can one's value be determined by who she marries and how can one think that all a woman has got to do is marry an "ok" man who can take care of her? And who even made men financiers? It is time for the society and even ourselves to re-evaluate the aspect of a woman's life we put value on- it should never be marriage! Marriage is never a career. Let's stop reducing our women's worth to a piece of jewellery- are they not worth more than that?

Why does the society hail men for what they have accomplished but women for who they are married to? And this is not limited to any society but most societies in the world. We belittle the abilities of women and define the totality of a woman by whoever she settles with. So a man born of a woman now shows the worth of a woman? This is so sickening. At least most men have grown very supportive and open-minded and they rather seek women who have wonderful careers and independent and not ones who feel their whole worth depends on a union. Marriage is never a career so don't sit there with your legs crossed waiting for someone's son who saw career as most important and worked at it before considering settling down or wouldn't allow marriage to cut short his career to find you serious.

I get heart broken when I hear stories like, `my husband asked me to stop working because he can cater for me' so are you telling yourself that you threw away your career because your husband is insecure and is scared of competition? I believe that even Mark Zuckerberg who has more than enough money allows his wife to work. So you threw your career away for a piece of jewellery- have you considered the possibility of a break up and what your life will be after that? Today, we have so many mentally-challenged women in hospitals and on the streets due to such situations. I personally know of one of such women who quit her nursing profession because her husband asked her to and got divorced by her husband later. She couldn't bear the situation because of all her sacrifices and she is on the streets today. Don't get carried away by the love of the moment to make certain decisions because even though marriage makes couples one, you too are still two different entities whose worth will be according to what you individually have achieved. Isn't it so lovely to be a supportive and working wife who shares the bill with your husband to ease him off several things? Isn't it lovely to be a wife who is financially sound to equally spoil your husband with gifts just as he does to you? Isn't it lovely as a wife to allow your husband to take a seat sometimes so you run the show? Some of these things kill the pressure and tension in marriages and even strengthens the bond.

I have this couple as neighbours and it is appalling how they are at each other's throat every time. The woman suffers a lot of domestic violence and all sorts of abuse from her husband all because she reduced her life to a piece of jewellery and sacrificed everything. She is not working and the husband alone takes care of their five children and sometimes he vents his frustration on her by beating her up and mistreating her knowing very well that she can't quit the marriage because she has nothing to survive on. Meanwhile, it was this same man who asked her to stop working in the early stages of their marriage and since she was carried away by the love at the moment, she couldn't think right. My dear sisters, marriage is good because it is good to find someone who loves you upon all your imperfections and want to be with you but please, it is not a career. Don't abandon your dreams for marriage. Pursue your career and that won't hinder you from getting married.

In the ancient times, women were primarily housewives and getting married was the real deal and the end goal- then, a woman was defined by her marriage and so, if you had no husband, you were not regarded a woman but this is no longer the case. In today's society, ladies are balancing much more than just finding a man or a husband. Today, women are entrepreneurs, CEOs, inventors, designers, pilots, engineers, captains, writers, teachers, and much more. Most women are walking out of the "marry after first degree and you are fulfilled" to getting their masters, doctorate degrees and etc. women are endlessly working to climb up the corporate ladder, women are in government, the law courts, changing the world with innovation, in fact women are everywhere so why must you see marriage as the real deal or end goal that is never to say that don't marry but that is to tell you that Marriage is not the end goal, it doesn't take you to Maslow's last stage on the pyramid, it is not a reason to abandon your career, it is not a Career.

Nothing can complete human, not even another human and that makes marriage no different- marriage like everything else like career, wealth, and etc can still never complete humans. Humans are insatiable. Love is sweet and so is marriage but it's ones own choice to get a life partner but it is always better when you are two- It takes two to tango.

There are a lot of successful career women out there who have wonderful marriages and are lovely wives and mothers- you don't need to sacrifice anything. You just need to make up your mind to reach to your dreams and be successful.

CHAPTER THREE-

NEVER SETTLE FOR LESS THAN YOU DESERVE

When you know your worth, you never settle for less. When you realize that you are a shark, a bait of worm will mean nothing to you. Most at times, we settle for less because we don't really know what we are worth. We let others take us for granted and belittle our capabilities because we don't know what we are worth. You know you have a good Curriculum Vitae (CV) and you deserve this job so why should you fall for the bargain of sleeping with the boss before getting it. He knows you are worth the job but he wants to know if you truly know your worth by asking for your body before he can employ you. Immediately you give in, he realizes that you don't really know your worth at that instance, he takes advantage of you. You are a great actress and you believe your great acting skills can earn you a role in any movie but once again, you don't know your worth and so you agree to sleep with the producer just to get a role you both know that you deserve. Most at times, it takes us to know our worth before we can decide never to settle for less. Until you do this, people will continue to take you for granted.

Your choices determine your value so never settle for less than you deserve. This applies to everything in life. If you consider yourself a person of high value, which you should, then you should set a high standard for yourself and who you associate with. Once you set a standard for yourself, you can expect only the best from yourself and the people around you. This is the recipe for success: building a life of high quality and never settling for less. You don't need to be pretty, rich, or connected to have a choice. No matter where you fall, never settle for less than you deserve.

You don't have to continue staying in that abusive relationship because you feel you can't be without him. Please, you must love yourself first and know your worth and when you do, no one can ever take you for granted. You don't have to rush into that marriage you never wished for because society is putting pressure on you. You just don't have to accept just any offer because you think you won't have any again. When you know who you are and your worth, you don't just settle for anything- you never settle for less than you deserve.

BELIEVE IN YOURSELF

You don't need anyone to believe in you, you must believe in yourself first before others can believe in you. When you have a high self-esteem and great confidence, you believe in yourself and you don't just settle for anything- you don't settle for less when you believe in yourself. The moment you decide to settle for less, you reduce your value. Have you wondered why people can't bargain at the mall for the reduction of prices but can do so in a normal market surrounding? Because, products in the mall are well packaged and shelved in confidence and a high self-esteem- most people think they are of quality and worth the higher price and will never complain but it's the exact opposite in the normal market setting. That should tell you that your composure will tell people who you are and what you are worth. Define yourself, rate yourself higher, and never settle for less by believing in yourself.

RESPECT YOURSELF

Respect, they say is reciprocal- until you respect yourself first as a person and know what to do and what not to do, no one will respect you. We don't force people to respect us, our actions inform that. When you lose respect, anything and anyone at all can take you for a ride because you lose your value and you are forced to settle for less.

AIM FOR PERFECTION

Never expect to achieve perfection but never give up in your pursuit of achieving perfection or that perfect life. If you set high standards for yourself, your achievements will be satisfactory and your rewards will be greater and outnumber your risks. If you are scared to fail, you will end up failing- you only need to see the perfection in failure and that is, it gives you the chance to try again and make better what you couldn't do earlier.

EMBRACE CHANGE

It is only a pessimist that is scared of change- embracing change is part of any optimistic person's agenda. You either see it as inevitable or settle for less than you deserve. It is your own choice to make, so call your shots. Oftentimes, we have a bad habit of accepting things in our lives that aren't necessarily good for us or are holding us back because we feel we can't do without them. This is a trait of one with a low self-esteem or self-confidence. You must filter out inferior things from your life in order to make room for what is truly great. Don't say, "I am holding on to this for a while" because you may never be able to do away with it. Don't hold on with anything, don't occupy yourself with unnecessarily good things but instead, make room for the things you seek- the greater things.

PART FIVE

CONTRIBUTIONS FROM OTHER WOMEN

CHAPTER ONE

by

Miss Anita Asante

In this chapter, I want us to concentrate on our decisions as women, our priorities and determination to fight for what we truly want and believe in. It focuses on a story-line of a young girl, Ama who compromised on her future for family benefits. Many at times, we all find ourselves in this situation of which some are unavoidable. But my main focus is, WHAT HAPPENS AFTER THE FALL? There are a wide range of opportunities after the fall, don't remain on the ground. This chapter will teach you how to make choices, love yourself, deal with abuse and rediscover and move on afterwards. It is specially dedicated to women who have been victims of abuse, no matter which form it came in.

Before the chapter begins I want you to believe in yourself and your capabilities. I want you to believe that you are sensational, bold, kind, fearless, resilient, wise, daring, courageous, virtuous, elegant, talented, breath taking, unique and wise.

MAKING CHOICES.

Ama bangs the door and runs outside. Walking away from all the drama seemed

easy. "You are going to marry Richard. He has it all. What do you need that degree for? He's going to take care of you well" her father's voice re-echoed.

Scenarios like these are very common in our societies. Situations where we are forced to hold on to marriage as a lifeline or as Mercedes Rowe Asamani will say, `as a career.' Women have been forced in many instances to neglect their dreams in exchange for a happy home. But the question is, when did success and hard work become a hindrance to a happy family? To me, such ideologies only come from either a woman who has lost their vision or basically men who are not emotionally strong enough to see their spouses successful- those who are intimidated by the success of women. It is said that what frightens men who are extremists most is a girl with books from which springs knowledge. Most men go to the extreme of stating that the Bible or Quran supports the submission of women. They however forget the price they have to pay for the submission- LOVE. A man who loves his wife would never let her forsake her dreams. Many women have gone through great ordeals in marriages and even love relationships because they thought they didn't need certificates or jobs to make a family work or possibly because they have been made to believe they were the responsibilities of men. But Michelle Obama states it clearly for us. "Success is only meaningful and enjoyable if it feels like your own". In our societies, many women live with the myth that a woman's success turns men off. Successful women especially celebrities have to deal with blames that their success is the reason for their singleness. They fail to see how easily though a passion, education or career can save them a lot of trouble by driving the wrong men away.

Women in our societies need to make a conscious effort to know themselves and be consistent in making choices. They should be ready to stand by their choices and take full responsibility of it despite criticisms and persuasions. They should make choices concerning their education or career and pursue it with all seriousness.

LOVING YOURSELF.

Two years into the marriage, Ama becomes a skeleton of herself. : Dependent on her man for everything and always home taking care of the house. She could barely talk to her children or husband. She felt she had failed herself, and the overwhelming guilt of it kept killing her gradually. She was shattered.

"Love thy neighbour as thyself" (Mark 12:31). Research shows that people who are happy and have strong affection for others are positive minded people who love themselves without reason. Note that the Bible said "as thyself" not more than yourself; not any lesser or greater than yourself. To be able to extend love to others you must be capable of loving yourself. Most women who have had to sacrifice their passion for petty reasons develop a sense of bitterness and guilt over time. There are instances when some women have become abusive to people around them, playing the blame game with them and developing hatred for others especially other women who have been able to make it. The accumulation of such negative energies leads to a life of hatred and even medical complications like mental sickness in extreme cases. Today's women must be taught to love themselves, be successful and proud of themselves before extending such love to others, whether your children, husband, business partners and friends. They must appreciate their talents and gifts, capabilities and the beauty of life. They must seek greater knowledge to understand themselves and the world around them. They must be made to endure the fall, failures, shortcomings and disappointments. They must understand that at a point in time they must be crushed, broken, abandoned and even loose themselves so that at the end they can rise, thrive, appreciate and above all love themselves.

"Love yourself first and everything else falls into line. You really have to love yourself to get anything done in this world" (Lucille Ball).

DEALING WITH ABUSE.

Ama sits on the parlour, facing her dad for the first time after her marriage. She

hadn't had the chance to visit him after the wedding since she was told by her

husband he was too busy for vacations and she was never given the opportunity

to go alone. It had been two years of constant pain and anguish and she really needed him now. "You have to make the family work again. He couldn't have just hit you

without a reason. Maybe you did something wrong, quickly apologize when he comes home." Ama burst out into tears. This was the last thing she needed now.

"A house where a woman is unsafe is not a home". (Unknown Author). Women worldwide have condoned abuse over centuries. These abuses come in various forms such as physical which is popularly known, emotional or even verbal. Much of the emotional and verbal abuse occur in forms of insult, constant discouragement or another person forcing a sense of guilt on your conscience making you feel belittled or unworthy as in Ama's case. Many endure this abuse with reasons such as the society's perception on divorce, protecting the children in the marriage or dependency on the man. Whichever form the abuse comes in, no woman must be a victim. Some men try to use these abuse strategies to show their superiority over the opposite gender but they must understand that nothing is weaker as compared to a man who hurts his family. True men drop their egos to help grow their women. Also, we have to understand that children in the family emulate or are affected by the examples we set at home. Most children become abusive to their mates because they have witnessed forms of abuses in the house. If women want to really protect the children, then it will be in their best interest to quit the marriage or relationship. Salma Hayek states and I quote, "No woman has to be a victim of physical abuse. Women have to feel like they are not alone". There are many institutions which can help solve such abusive cases. Report the matter to an authority. Forget the `so you are getting your husband arrested' and `think of the kids' reporters. They were nowhere close when you were being abused. Don't be intimidated that he will have to spend some few years in prison or the marriage will break up,

113

that's the price he pays for his choices. Stand up for yourself and your children if any. Break free. Be confident and bold. Make a choice to be happy and break yourself away from abuse. You will be doing yourself a lot of good.

REDISCOVERING YOURSELF AND MOVING ON.

She laid down on the hospital bed, thinking of the events of the past few weeks.

As usual her abusive husband had hit her and this time she had lost her third child and almost her life in the incidence. The hospital authorities had convinced her to make it a legal case and she had agreed. Her husband had been arrested and testimonies from her previous abuse had landed him three years in jail. What was she going to do now? How was she going to survive?

So he left, what now? How do you go on with your life? Yes I understand your world revolved around him. You spent majority of your time doing his bidding so you are scared to move on without him. He was your pillar and now the society is stigmatizing you for being the woman who got her husband arrested. What is the next step forward?

Moving on with your life after an abusive relationship can be quite difficult and stressful. It requires a lot of energy and self-determination. Most women breakdown during the process because it requires a conscious effort to erase memories of the past and starting a new life as if nothing happened. However, Guy Finley says, "Nothing in the universe can stop you from letting go and starting over" and as it is always said "it's better to be alone than to be with someone who makes you feel alone". To be able to do this you need to rediscover yourself. You need to ask yourself some basic questions. 'Who are you?' The most important question you can ask yourself. You need to delve into your innermost soul to answer this. Your purpose in life, who you want to be, things you love to do, what makes you happy and what keeps you going. Mostly, taking a vacation helps a lot. Move away from the noise, stress, anger, struggles and negativity. During this period you can find a confidant to talk to. A therapist, counsellor, friend, family, anyone, provided they can be trusted. Keeping the pain in you wouldn't help. Let it out, talk to someone. Your next step is to forgive. It's the hardest process but you must go through. Keeping grudges only wounds the heart deeper. See it as a stepping stone to progress. Free your mind and soul. Now my favourite part, Enjoy yourself. Choose something fun to do. M. Kathleen Casey states, "Pain is inevitable but suffering is optional". A party, picnic with friends, writing, arts, singing, traveling, anything you find fun to do, do it. Laugh at the world, help the needy or join a volunteer group in the society. Remember, making others happy automatically brings you happiness. A little advice from Elizabeth Taylor; She says, "Pour yourself a drink, put on some lipstick and pull yourself together".

114

So the vacation is over, you are free to go, what next? I would say, Start Building Again. Set goals and objectives. Set a time limit to achieve those goals. Work hard towards it and be good at it. Have a lot of self-respect for the woman you are becoming. Raise yourself above the waters and specialize in your field of interest. Don't rush into another relationship just yet. Give yourself time to fully heal. After understanding yourself try to understand others. Why they do what they do, how they feel, their perception about life, how they do things and the external motives behind their actions. This way you will expect less from people and wouldn't be hurt or disappointed by their decisions. After building that trust with yourself and others, I think you are ready to move on.

Everyone deserves a second chance. Wait! I am not talking about that abusive partner. I am referring to you. Yes, YOU. Give yourself another chance to love. Don't close your heart to love. Don't build a wall around you. Find love again and this time make it right. Find someone who supports your dreams and visions. You might have a kingdom at this stage so find someone you can turn it into an empire with. Look for someone who would appreciate and love your kids, if you have any. Settle with someone you can confidently open up to about your past so that he can find better ways of loving you. He should be able to understand your struggles so that he can admire your success. Clear the `all men are the same' notion and treat him right, settle down and have a family again. Until such a man pops up, keep your panties up and concentrate on being more successful. Nothing shines brighter than gold which went through the worst inferno.

Always keep in mind that Beyond the Clitoris is a wide range of opportunities and power, achievements and glory, love and success. Be Bold, take a step today.

115

CHAPTER TWO-

by

Mrs. Grace Afia Larbi

PREGNANCY/CHILDLESSNESS IN OUR SOCIETY

Pregnancy which leads to childbirth (if all goes well) is a blessing or gift that God Almighty gave to man as a means of procreation, hence He asked us to be fruitful and multiply. As God's representatives on earth He enables us to recreate, albeit, a bit differently from how He did it.

Pregnancy as a process usually comes with its own package for the mother-to-be. Like life itself, some have it smooth like a cruise from conception through to birth, while others have it real rough like a rough ride on the Salaga road. Yet, others too would usually have a mixed package. Indeed so many things do come into play: hormones which affect the emotions, psyche, physical and total being of the mother; or vice versa.

In the African society, pregnancy and childbirth are held in such high esteem to the extent that even in these modern times, couples can be under that much pressure if after a year of marriage there's not a sign of pregnancy. In all of this the woman mostly bears the brunt of it all. She is able and truly able to pull through if she has the man's total support and the man does not succumb to the pressure in any way.

In our society, when a young unmarried lady gets pregnant, it is considered an abomination, and hence teenage (`child') pregnancy is so frowned upon. Again, depending on their family status or background, some of these young ladies usually go in for abortions.

Huh! - That one- abortion! We are safe as a society only if they would muster courage and see professional doctors and not quack ones for the procedure. Worse still is when they themselves make attempts at this by using crude methods such as; Guinness and sugar solution, consumption of strong local spirit (akpeteshie), etc.

Some young girls tend to have supportive families and very principled parents too and do not allow abortions no matter the circumstances. If such young girls are fortunate, their education is deferred for the period and are made to return to the classroom after childbirth, while their parents/ family take care of the child. Indeed there are several such examples who have made it in life and are worthy of emulation.

Yet again, the other side of the coin is somewhat interesting. When a young couple is expected within a year of marriage to have a child and there's no signal, eyebrows are raised. When it prolongs then `wahala' (trouble) brews. In the same vein as pre-marital pregnancy is frowned upon in our society, so is marriage without children.

Let me share my personal experience. I married rather late by societal standards, a couple of months from hitting thirty years; especially when my sister, born after me, had married at twenty-three `pronto' and already had two children of her own. Well, fast forward ten years, we're patiently still waiting. Has it been easy? - No! Were eyebrows raised? - Yes! So some one year plus the line, the questions started. Genuine as some were, others were with lots of inhibitions and criticisms. Those seem quite easy and `ignorable' but when the real pressure mounted from all sides, with snide remarks (the akan will say `akutia') were coming in, I almost broke down! But thanks to a supportive family and husband's support and firmness, and above all the Almighty God for his words of assurances now and then; I guess I would not have had that much courage to be part of social functions, especially ones that had to do with babies. The issue of delays in childbirth or lack of childbirth can be medical, psychological, and/or even spiritual. It could stem from either spouse, yet is not interesting to note that more often than not, women are blamed and seen as culprits in this regard?

So what? Well there is light at the end of the tunnel. Indeed I have read about, seen and met couples who have been blessed with children at latter parts of their lives when they least expected and almost given up.

Society is and will always be ready to mount the pressure but hardly ever ready to support; whether physically, financially, emotionally or psychologically. But let us as individuals, be more than prepared as couples, especially we the women, hopefully with supportive husbands to stand firm in such trying times; for life in itself comes with all sorts of challenges. This is but one of them. Trust me, this is just an inexhaustible and I could go on forever, tackling from more perspectives, but hey I made my point.

Personally, I pray for couples especially when they marry afresh that they be blessed with the joy of children quickly. I also counsel and give encouragement to those whom I know, and ask them to trust the perfect will of Our Father in Heaven.

Let me leave you with a scenario. A friend lost his wife after childbirth after waiting for nine solid years (hey I know you have gone beyond that) for one. He just said, much as it was the doctor's negligence, and the family lawyer was willing to take the doctor on, it wasn't going to change the fact that she was gone. But what really got me thinking was another thing he said. He said he believed God saw it coming, so maybe He should have kept His child up there and he would still have had his wife. This is not to scare us, but to end God knows best and His perfect will will be done and will be done always!

My final word in addition to this is yes, let's do all the needed medical checks by all means, but in all of it let's not lean on our own understanding but trust in God to direct our paths; or trust in the arm of flesh, having faith that His perfect will is accomplished.

Effie Sam *(Pen Name), January 26, 2017.*

MARRIAGE

According to Wikipedia, marriage, also called matrimony or wedlock, is a socially or ritually recognized union between spouses that establishes rights and obligations between them, between them and their children, and between them and their in-laws. The definition of marriage varies according to different cultures, but it is principally an institution in which interpersonal relationships, usually sexual, are acknowledged. In some cultures, marriage is recommended or considered to be compulsory before pursuing any sexual activity. When defined broadly, marriage is considered a universal culture.

Some people marry for several reasons, including legal, social, libidinal, emotional, financial, spiritual, and religious purposes. Their choice of partners is usually influenced by societal rules of incest, prescriptive marriage rules, parental choice and individual desire. In some parts of the world, arranged marriage, child marriage, polygamy, and sometimes forced marriage, may be practiced as a cultural tradition. Conversely, such practices may be outlawed and penalized in parts of the world out of concerns for women's rights and on the basis of international law. In developed parts of the world, there has been a general trend towards ensuring equal rights within marriage for women and legally recognizing the marriages of interfaith or interracial, and same-sex couples. These trends coincide with the broader human rights movement.

Marriage is recognized by a state, an organization, a religious authority, a tribal group, a local community or peers; hence the different types of marriage such as civil marriage, or the one in a religious setting via a wedding ceremony. Marriage has normative or legal obligations between the individuals involved, and any offspring they may produce. In terms of legal recognition, most sovereign states and other jurisdictions limit marriage to opposite-sex couples; though scantily we come across some that permit polygyny, child marriages, and forced marriages. Over the twentieth century, a growing number of countries and other jurisdictions have lifted bans on and have established legal recognition for interracial marriage, interfaith marriage, and most recently, gender-neutral marriage.] Some cultures allow the dissolution of marriage through divorce or annulment. In some areas, child marriages and polygamy may occur in spite of national laws against the practice.

Marriage over the period has had its own fair share of controversies with regards to especially the woman's role and rights among others. In the 21st century, some controversies persists, regarding the legal status of married women, legal acceptance of or leniency towards violence

118

within marriage (especially sexual violence), traditional marriage customs such as dowry and bride price, forced marriage, marriageable age, and criminalization of consensual behaviours such as premarital and extramarital sex.

You realize that so far I have said nothing practically but giving definitions, with trends and instances. Well, all of the above said, I believe strongly that marriage is a beautiful thing, an institution well established by the Almighty God at creation. (Genesis 1:27; 2:23-24 - The Holy Bible). However, human as we are, we have always found ways to adulterate (in some cases, destroy) what our Creator did. God did not plan for divorce to be in the picture, yet the rate is on the ascendancy. But this came about because the Israelites were `stubborn' and Moses granted it and it was established.

Marriage like life itself, needs working at and guess what, most couples assume getting married is the end result and/or believe they have arrived. Rather, it is the beginning of a project together, where both partners will have to jaw-jaw. They will have to agree on some terms and goals to work with. They will have to discuss and plan their lives with some goals in mind. It's a whole journey of partnership. And oh! Like any partnership, there may be disagreements on pertinent issues till all the fine tunings are done. And even then, as a friend of mine puts it: it is a lifetime of learning new things everyday about your partner. We got to have the will power to let it work.

That notwithstanding, if you happen to be in a relationship that is abusive by all standards, please move out first before resolving issues. Sometimes, just sometimes we need out to be able to get back in permanently.

I will like to share my almost a decade experience. Like the wedding cake, mine has been sweet and sour, has had its fair share of ups and downs and the struggle of responsibilities. We went in there together telling ourselves we have just us and we were willing to work through it. We discussed many issues from lack of childbirth or delays, extra marital affairs, finances, our spiritual life and life's general issues; coming to the same page on these issues after several talks and hearty discussions (some moments in discussing these were not so comfortable though). So we took it one day at a time. First the euphoria and incredulity of being married didn't wear off us easily; and I must say till date some people who meet us for the first time, mostly don't believe we have been married for almost a decade now. Well that is grace. Our first marital disagreement was, in hindsight trivial now and very funny. So we both love cereals very much and we had a tin of Cerelac always for a quick fix and convenience sake when needed. Well on one occasion I got home rather famished and needed a quick fix before getting the main meal ready. Warm water in cup and ready for my fix, I opened the tin of Cerelac, took a couple of spoons only to realize it was gari (flaked cassava)! Whatever happened to the Cerelac?! My husband had taken it raw in the evening while watching movies; knowing I would be upset, he chose not to mention it at all, hoping I would not notice too soon. That started a fight and if I remember well we didn't talk to each other for a couple of days till it was replaced. There have been other major misunderstanding, where suddenly we felt like we didn't understand each other and we wanted out. What he always say when we had an argument was, "well I know you feel like you want out, but I'm sorry young lady, there's no way out. We're confined within these four walls and you stuck with me so keep calm." It could really upset me. There were times we took vacation apart from each other to clear our heads. Sometimes it worked and sometimes it didn't. There was always a way around it once God was in control. But through it all we let love; respect for each and our relationship with God take precedence.

We wore different caps to communicate. (We were each other's ten-in-one e.g. brother/sister, daddy/mummy and friend role, among others). It made communication easier. We also kept the third party out mostly, though we could speak to trusted buddies individually. The idea here was not to seek advice per se but to have a friend to talk to, vent all the emotions, etc. (NB: very important to have an electric pole - a trusted friend you can express yourself well with). The issue of planning your careers, your finances and being a team is key in all you do. We made sure to always come to win-win conclusion in all situations, and we dialogued till we got to a satisfying point for both of us.

I could really go on and on, but that will be another story for another time (or see me in chambers). I would conclude here that marriage is a beautiful institution, yet like life itself, it has its own ups and downs. Our attitude in there, our selflessness and our dependence on God, will make all the difference. So far I have enjoyed my marriage and I trust God to enable me continue enjoying it and letting God's will be done in there!

SOCIETAL MISCONCEPTIONS

Doesn't our entire world have loads of misconceptions about lots of things?! I will in this write up, limit myself to misconceptions about women. The initial role of women was solely domestic, where they had no voice, no vote, and no say.

In spite of great achievements towards gender equality (I prefer to call it equity) in this century, women are still subjected to negative labels, double standards and impossible binds by a world that in some ways, seems to have moved beyond rigid gender roles, yet at the same time still imprison women to the past; considering that women form half of the workforce and population. Despite many years of progress in many respects, women are still held to the restrictive rules and roles that pertained long ago.

One particular and quite popular example is a young budding lady or a woman in her prime who is working at/has achieved great laurels in academics/career, and is not in any `serious' relationship or marriage. I remember when some of my friends were getting married in their early twenties and I was gradually hitting my thirties and seem to be more focused on my career and furthering education, my Grandma would always ask," When ooo when". Though we laughed over it and she still encouraged me, somewhere in my subconscious, it always rang a bell. She personally wasn't much perturbed but she was aligning with the societal norm that as the first Granddaughter she didn't want other relatives to be bad mouthing me. As much as in her own way she felt she was protecting me from `bad mouthing', but I still felt the pressure in a subtle way.

Society generally believes that a woman's happiness and fulfillment is ultimately in marriage, but we all know that marriage is not necessarily the means to happiness or fulfillment. They forget that it is not a means to an end. They forget it can be a matter of choice based on certain experiences and issues. Marriage doesn't automatically take away issues of insecurity and loneliness. Sometimes at a certain age/caliber society wants to judge you as being too picky with your choice hence your singleness. They equally forget that being single is neither a cocktail party nor prison.

Another side of it is once you hit your forties the suggestions of having a child or two while unmarried comes into play. Again society frowns on you judgmentally, assuming you didn't do something right that's why you are without family. No one thinks that you could have been widowed early without child. No one is thinking of some traumatic experience that may have scarred you for life.

Also, with regards to professional advancement or moving up the ladder, more often than not, society will not just applaud but will equally murmur that you slept your way up (Something I find real sad and very disheartening); or with the ideology that women cannot lead.

Some men equally have certain misconceptions or stereotypes about women. They assume all women are the same in all regards and want the same thing; so they tend give all women the same treatment, irrespective of the environment they find themselves in. They assume all women are irrationally emotional, lack good sense of humour and love to play games, just to test them. They also believe that women/girls are not good at Science and Math, because it is a man's world and women crack under pressure. More so, some even perceive women's empowerment as detrimental to men.

In the same vein, due to some of these misconceptions and stereotyping, women have been abused physically, emotionally and psychologically. Society is always quick to point women out as having one form of witchcraft or the other, being camped in isolation and yet, may I ask; how many men have been accused of such or been isolated?

Even when a woman is sexually abused she is definitely at fault. She either asked for it by her dressing, mood, attitude, etc. Even when she says `no', she is being tagged as playing `hard to get'.

Indeed I could go on forever, but I would conclude that in all of this motherhood is regarded by society as the quintessential accomplishment of a woman.

CHAPTER THREE-

by

Abena Magis-Gatugbe

REALITIES OF LOVE

When I was young, I didn't understand why some women allowed themselves to get into the sort of situations they did.

Questions I asked myself were:

Why endure pain and suffering all because you say you love a man?

Why put kids into situations where all they see is your pain and strife which could affect them all their lives?

But I've grown up to realize that it's not just based on the woman's emotional needs at that time but also on the circumstances they find themselves in.

Ama moved to stay in Nigeria with her husband. They had 3 kids. She had tried to get a job several times but wasn't successful so her husband told her to be a house wife. He was gainfully employed and could cater for them without her having to add a kobo. 15 years of a relatively wealthily lived life passed by and her husband died. When he did, he left behind unpaid debts and a bank loan which had to be serviced with the very house they lived in. So left koboless after her husband's demise, she had no option than to call back home and plead for help.

She returned to Ghana with a fridge, standing fan and clothes. Her kids were understandably devastated but she more so because of the ridicule she was subjected to by some family members who had secretly envied her easy life in another country and now having to part away with money and time to make her feel "loved."

Now the question begging to be asked is why did she put herself in such a situation? Her husband had money, true. She couldn't get a job when she went job hunting but why didn't she still press on or become an entrepreneur by starting a project of her own say a convenient store or something? Why did she get so comfortable?

Now instead of looking at things at face value, let's go back to Ama's story.

Ama and her husband moved to Nigeria in 1978. That was the era when Nigerians were employing a lot of Ghanaians to teach them most particularly English. Unfortunately a lot of head teachers wanted only male teachers. She was a trained teacher and met some of such head teachers. She visited a lot of schools and had to give up her job search over this. She found herself pregnant in 1980, gave birth in 1981 and decided to wait till her child was around 2 years before looking for jobs again. In 1983, when her girl was 2 years, the Nigerian president Shehu Shagari suddenly announced and gave all foreigners without the right paperwork a few weeks to leave the country.

A majority of these immigrants were from Ghana. "If they don't leave they should be arrested and tried and sent back to their homes. Illegal immigrants, in fact, under normal circumstances, should not be given any notice whatsoever," an official statement from Nigerian authorities announced.

Ama's husband had been able to secure his paperwork and so was free to work but not his wife. She had no option than to stay at home and hope that no one will come home one day, find her there and forcefully sack her or worse, kill her like some thugs had been doing.

The expulsion lasted for some months but by the time some Ghanaians started returning back to Nigeria almost a year later, Ama found she was pregnant again. She had to wait again for some years before thinking of job hunting. Her husband who had always lived in fear of coming home and not finding her or worse, killed, warned her not to step out unless he was with her. She had to take care of their kids. He was making good money and could take care of all of them.

She went on to give birth to a third child and with 3 children having various growing needs, she gave up all her ambitions and rather focused on being the best wife and mother she could be. That's what got her in the situation she found herself in years later.

Like Ama, there are so many times women find themselves in situations they had never imagined themselves to be in. It is only after they are no longer in that situation that they will during a post mortem analysis of the situation ask themselves why they allowed themselves to go through it all.

My mum and dad were married for 17 years before they divorced. It was a marriage riddled with domestic abuse, cheating, she having to take care of him for years while he was job hunting among other situations. People knew my dad was cheating on her. She found him in bed with another woman when I was 4 and caught him doing same over and over again. She was physically abused with belts and even furniture but she still stayed. When I was 16, she asked for a divorce and he readily gave it to her.

Anyone reading to her story would ask, why wait till your child is 16 before asking for divorce? I was 2 years away from being 18. I was in SSS at that time so wasn't the divorce going to affect me? What about my younger brother? Why hadn't she asked for it sooner or waited till say, I had finished SSS or even the university, after all, she had endured all these for 16 years?

Now, let's go back to my mother's story.

When my mum met my dad, he was this simple lad from the Volta Region and pursuing his first degree while she was working in a hospital. She is a Fante and any such union between Akans and Ewes was under more scrutiny than it is now. She enrolled in a nursing training school but unfortunately had to leave because she found herself pregnant, I was the foetus using her stomach as my football field at that time, and per the school's directive which disallowed pregnant women from schooling there, she had no option than to leave the school. She knew that if she still wanted to further her education, she would have to wait till I was born and then somehow find the money to go back to school.

During the 70s, one of the studios which had gained prominence in West Africa belonged to no other person than the late Fela Anikulapo Kuti. My dad had had aspirations of becoming a gospel musician and so he decided to follow the example of the highlife musician Nana Tuffour by going there to also record.

He traveled to Nigeria with my pregnant mum and she gave birth to me in Fela's house. My dad became one of Fela's guitarists but his dreams were thwarted a few years later when the `Ghana must go' exodus began. My parents had no option than to go to Benin and take a boat from there to Ghana.

When they reached, Ghana was battling a severe famine caused by a yearlong drought. With the influx of Ghanaians from Nigeria, getting a job was tough. Thankfully after 2 years, my father landed a job at Saint Augustine's College and from there went back to UCC to pursue his masters. My mother was able to get her old job back and also had to deal with the birth of my little brother.

Now that they had finally settled, my mum had to endure finding out that my dad had brought in a second wife in the guise of a nanny. When she found out, I was 5 and my brother just some months old. She had no option than to still stay in her marriage and be the first wife.

There were a series of unrests in UCC and my dad was sacked because it was believed that he had initiated them. He was given a period within which to vacate the premises allocated to him so my mum had to send money to her relatives to finish building my grandmother's part of the family house so we could move in. My mother at that time had wanted to further her education but these had to be pushed aside because my dad was now jobless. The only employed spouse was my mom and so she had no option than to cater for her family while following a heavy work schedule.

When my dad finally got a job and started working, my mum decided to continue her schooling. My dad decided to get married to another woman and for a woman who had had to go through his years of cheating and domestic abuse, that was too much for her to handle. She asked him to choose and he chose my step mother. End of their marriage.

I look at both stories and it's obvious that these are women who could have changed their circumstances if they could but couldn't.

We have all fallen for or will fall for men who will hurt us. Years later, we will look back and wonder why we allowed ourselves into such situations. It will obviously be based on the circumstances we find ourselves in and our mindsets.

I fell deeply in love with one of my best friends. I was 19 years at that time. We were both naturally shy but obviously not to each other. I later broke up with him because I thought he didn't love me. Years later, I looked back at the circumstances behind our being together and our subsequent break up and all I could put it down to is that the circumstances in which we fell in love didn't favour us.

How we relate with our partners, permeates every aspect of our lives.

Women because of our empathetic nature have had to sacrifice either family to become a career woman or sacrificed our career for our family's sake. It has been hard balancing this especially if we have little or no support from our men.

A lot of people ask me that why do I use the hashtag #ManoKekaMe and talk so much on relationships when there are so many topics I could dwell on. Some have wondered why I don't channel my passion into politics fully or follow notable courses than to talk about relationships all the time.

I have and will always say that, a woman can never be who she wants to be if her relationships don't allow her. How many women haven't harmed themselves, gone insane or just given up in life because of relationships? These are women who would have contributed immensely to our country if their relationships hadn't gotten in the way of whatever aspirations they had.

I have with all the stories shared on my Realities of Love page realized that when women get affected by relationship issues, they mostly become reactive than proactive. They are so focused on enduring that they push any thoughts of finding solutions away.

I believe it is time women entered into relationships with laid down plans of what to do when certain situations come up. They must from the very onset of the relationship plan how to marry their personal needs, family pressures, work and relationship needs. They must also make contingency plans should anything happen because when their relationships fail, it will as it has happened for Millennia, affect every aspect of her life.

CHAPTER FOUR-

by

Agbenyo Delali Rhoda

I AM ABLE.

I have not been raped before, I have never been heart broken; neither have I been at the receiving end of unrequited love and I definitely haven't experienced financial crisis pushing me to go against my principles. I really admire such strong people. Despite discouragement here and there, they made it. But I have had my share of unfavourable incidents, one of which I share with you.

Have you ever been in a situation where people doubted your abilities, it pissed you off so much that you gave it a try to prove to yourself and the world that you are able? Have you ever been discriminated against because of your gender, race and stature? I have lived my whole 2 decades and counting on earth being doubted. Doctors doubted I would live to clock my first year of birth. My parents were made to believe I would not survive an illness I contracted a few months after my birth. To make matters worse, when all hope was lost, I spoke my first word. My daddy who couldn't take it anymore cried. He said " She has even started speaking and I am about to lose her". But here I am today telling you a story with more than a word. That explains why I am a talker. My God is wonderful.

Once I am told a feat is impossible for me to attain, I am gingered to prove that person wrong. I go the extra mile to break that stereotype. This earned me a lot of names, I achieved these things just to spite people. Then, I realized those people do not matter. They have no say in how I run my life. I have my sanity to protect. I owe them no apology with how I live. I need not be coerced to do things because they say so.

As a requirement for Senior High School, I went for a prospectus to prepare for school. People-teachers and students- thought I had accompanied my elder sister to school. It was shocking to see a tiny girl who would easily pass for a 10-year-old primary student there. The day of arrival was pretty much the same, it's just that lots of people witnessed the scene. 'Sisters' tried to intimidate the ' un-intimidatable'. They assumed my stature was proportional to my courage and saw it as an opportunity to scare me. But I made them understand that a book should not be judged by its cover. Things were not rosy. I had to adapt to new people, new environment while combating illnesses. I spent half of my senior high school days in hospitals and home, while my colleagues were learning. My parents, my mother especially, were scared. "Would she leave that school alive?" "Did we make a mistake of sending her to school?" These questions and many more, my parents asked themselves every day. I was of the view that should my parents die, it will be out of hypertension due to frequent and incessant calls from unknown numbers informing them their daughter had been admitted at the hospital. Thankfully, they did not give up on me. I am who I am today because of their prayers, support, dedication and commitment.

This badly affected my academics. Which science student is almost always not in class, or had her head on the table when she is present? A Physics tutor asked me one day if I was fit to be in the Science class. She wondered if I would ever complete my three year stay in school as a science student. According to her, with the rate at which I fell sick, it would be impossible for me to complete the course. I understood that, as a caring mother, she thought I would have thrived in a more relaxed environment. At that moment, my resolve was strengthened more than ever. I was more than determined to make it in life. Today, I am still pursuing that dream. Every step gets me closer to that goal. Weak immune system or not, I will get to the top. And I wish to see you there.

Being a lady, I was told I can't do what men are allowed to do. I faced discrimination, yet I persevered. Today, I can boldly say my kid sisters have a model to look up to when they're told a lady can't do everything. Today, everyone, even my detractors, can testify that I Am Able. Hey, I do not assume I have arrived, I am getting there and so can you. I tell myself always, that I am Able. I am able, abundantly able to do what I set my heart to do. It may not look like I've overcome, but I'll surely get there.

Have you been discouraged by people around you? Do friends and family not believe in you? Hold on, do not be discouraged. You'll tell your story one day. Work till you get up there. I am not where I wish to be, not even half, but I know someone looks up to me for inspiration. I know someone would say if Rhoda can do it, then so can I. "Cannot" should not be in your dictionary. Once you know that venture is profitable, go for it. Those who discourage you today will blame you tomorrow for not trying.

You must realize that everyone gets discouraged sometimes. You're no exception. What would set you apart is if you let the discouragement discourage you from giving up. Whoever doesn't get discouraged is not human. Discouragements come and go. But an opportunity once missed is difficult to regain.

WHAT CAUSES DISCOURAGEMENTS?

FEAR

This four letter word is capable of annihilating a mighty man. We most times deny its presence, but hey, who are we kidding? Fear is the major cause of discouragement, accept it or not. The fear of failure, responsibility, stereotype, the society, prevents capable women, and men, from achieving their goals.

FAILURE

The most painful experience in life is failure. To fail a course; failure to move to the next phase of life. Just when you felt life is beginning to make sense, some unforeseen misfortunes confuse you the more. We all have been there before. The times when you fail and they say it's normal for a woman to fail, because she doesn't belong there. Or when they say, your inability to deliver is why they do not allow women hold certain positions. You're already working twice your male colleague to make the same impact they make.

FAMILY AND FRIENDS

Those we expect to incite us to make it in life are those who pull us down the most. Some have genuine concerns; others are there to prevent you from getting to the top. You must be able to discern between such people.

DISEASES

Diseases and deformities have the tendency to discourage individuals. It is worse when it is accompanied by taunts from people around that individual. They lose their confidence, coil into their shells and accept anything that comes their way.

HOW TO AVOID DISCOURAGEMENT

- **ACKNOWLEDGE THE PROBLEM**
  In my case, I admitted I had a problem. I realized I couldn't avoid being ill. This phase gives you an idea of what you are up against. When you know the problem, explore deeper. Ask necessary questions and solve it.

- **DONT SPEND TIME WITH PEOPLE WHO DISCOURAGE YOU**
  People, family and loved ones, attempt to discourage you. It is human nature. The best you can do is to avoid their company altogether. Being around them will make you reconsider your decision to undertake a worthy course. Do not knit your life around their failure stories. You are different. That they failed doesn't mean you would too. Take a cue from their mistakes and make it happen. It is better to lose friends than lose focus.

- **TAKE A BREAK**
  Taking a break does not make you weak. It gives you time to recuperate and prepare you for the task ahead. The danger here is you might stay here for longer days than necessary which can either discourage you the more or make you lose interest in your mission. It is good to rest. But remember to keep it brief. While you rest, recount your successes. Most times we capitalize on our problems and failures, belittling the victories. Write them down if you can, it will give you the strength to face the storms.

- **REMIND YOURSELF OF THE BENEFITS**
  You want to lose weight, but it's not going as expected? Remind yourself of what you stand to achieve after you see this project through. After you lose weight, you will be able to live healthy; chronic diseases like hypertension and diabetes stay away; you can fit into that dress you always dream of. Keep going. Always remind yourself of the end result and you will get there.

- **DO IT**
  It is action time. The only way to avoid being discouraged is to do it. You must know that that problem will always be there and in some cases become compounded if you don't solve it right away. Get up, dust yourself up and DO IT. Follow your heart. Be the best you can ever be and the rest will follow.

- PRAY
  Prayer is the key to lock or unlock all the problems you face. Believe it or not, God has the answers. Spend some time with him. Listen to him more than you grumble and he shall direct your path.

I will meet you at the top. I am taking life one day at a time. I know one day, I will look back and say, I am grateful I didn't give up.

Discover other title(s) by Mercedes Rowe Asamani:

- **Journey to the Polls** *(2016)*

Thank you for reading this book. This book is available in print at most online retailers.

PERSONAL NOTES:

PERSONAL NOTES:

PERSONAL NOTES:

PERSONAL NOTES: